Clinical Surgery MADE EASY

A companion to problem-based learning

Mohan de Silva

tfm Publishing Limited
Castle Hill Barns
Harley
Shrewsbury
SY5 6LX
UK

Tel: +44 (0)1952 510061
Fax: +44 (0)1952 510192
E-mail: nikki@tfmpublishing.com
Web site: www.tfmpublishing.com

Design & Typesetting: Nikki Bramhill BSc (Hons) Dip Law Solicitor

First Edition: September 2008, © 2008 tfm publishing Ltd.
Front cover image (left): © 1999 Image 100 Ltd.
Front cover image (background): © Comstock Inc., www.comstock.com

ISBN: 978 1 903378 65 6

Printed by Gutenberg Press Ltd., Gudja Road, Tarxien, PLA 19, Malta.

Tel: +356 21897037; Fax: +356 21800069.

FSC

Mixed Sources
Product group from well-managed forests, and other controlled sources
www.fsc.org Cert no. TT-CoC-002424
© 1996 Forest Stewardship Council

The paper used for this book is FSC-certified and totally chlorine-free. FSC (the Forest Stewardship Council) is an international network to promote responsible management of the world's forests.

Contents

Preface

Creating a differential diagnosis and rationalising a treatment plan is a challenging task for medical students at the early stage of their training. This process will also expose deficiencies in core knowledge and problems in applying certain components of their knowledge to varied clinical situations. Guided by experienced teachers, students best learn these skills at the bedside. Patients do not always present with classic textbook descriptions and clinical scenarios can be very varied. During the limited period of clinical training allocated to the surgical curriculum, students may not receive sufficient exposure to an evidence-based approach and decision making in clinical surgery. Medical schools with problem-based curricula rely heavily on clinical teachers and under their guidance, students are expected to present and discuss cases at clinical tutorials. There is evidence that problem-based learning (PBL) stimulates critical thinking. In addition to clinical exposure, PBL demands focused reading, commitment and enthusiasm to acquire the essential core knowledge pertinent to a topic and its application to varied clinical situations.

An alternative method of supplementing the bedside experience is to carefully design a series of common clinical scenarios in general surgery to simulate the clinical decision-making approach, and under each topic, to highlight the essential core knowledge and relevant clinical pathways. This approach will guide students to recognise, recall and apply the relevant facts to given clinical situations.

This book presents such an approach. Learning objectives are given at the commencement of each scenario. The essential components of clinical anatomy, pathophysiology, and the core knowledge pertinent to the topic are presented. The diagnostic and therapeutic approach based on the available guidelines (e.g. NICE, SIGN, BASO, BSG*) and frequently asked questions at examinations are emphasised during discussion. Clinically important points are reiterated in boxes for easy review. Self-assessment questions in the form of EMQs (Extended Matching Questions), SBAs (Single Best Answers) and True/False types with the relevant explanatory notes are included at the end of each topic. The questions are created to reinforce the concepts and to try to inspire the student's thirst for knowledge. Some questions are purposely created outside the parameters discussed, to stimulate the need for further reference on the topic.

The book is primarily aimed at undergraduates and junior doctors.

Professor Mohan de Silva MS, FRCS (Edin), Professor of Surgery
Faculty of Medical Sciences, University of Sri Jayawardenepura
Colombo, Sri Lanka and Honorary Consultant General Surgeon
Mid Cheshire Hospitals NHS Foundation Trust, UK

* (NICE - National Institute for Health and Clinical Excellence, SIGN - Scottish Intercollegiate Guidelines Network, BASO - British Association of Surgical Oncology, BSG - British Society of Gastroenterology).

Foreword

Standard textbooks can be daunting. This book is different. I believe that students will find this an easy read and will be able to translate the scenarios into an understanding of how clinical pathways are constructed. By asking questions through the pathways students are encouraged to develop their own ideas - a form of problem-based learning rather than learning by rote. Retention of facts is so much easier when they form part of a story.

The book is borne out of many years of Professor de Silva's teaching experience and the conducting of examinations for undergraduates and postgraduates. He has written in a style which demonstrates a form of 'thinking out loud', discussing the pros and cons for a particular decision, and providing bite-sized packets of information from evidence-based guidelines to produce a special and out of the ordinary learning tool.

Competent clinicians need to take an active interest in their patients. Undoubtedly the best stimulus is direct contact with patients in the clinical environment, following them through their medical journey, with enthusiastic help from senior colleagues. It is the clinical pictures which endure as memory that constitute 'experience'. With subspecialisation the opportunities for students to come into contact with a wide range of disease entities and variations of presentations are limited. Professor de Silva has written these case scenarios from the point of view of an enthusiastic teacher, stimulating his students to think through the pathways and in the process giving them confidence to attend clinics, wards and theatres. It is to be hoped that these activities will stimulate them to read in depth about the conditions that they encounter. His very wide experience of surgery in its generality, acute and elective, as well as specialised skills gained from his time in the UK and Sri Lanka, give him the perspective of the basic requirements for a practical understanding of the needs of students around the globe.

Additions of a series of questions at the end of each chapter are in the style of many examinations and familiarity with these is a vital part of preparation for examinations. Professor de Silva's book should help students to pass those examinations and equip the young doctor with an approach from which they can enjoy their clinical experience whilst at the same time benefiting their patients. The book can also be used as a 'refreshing' tool for continued medical education or as a simple guide book for practising clinicians dealing with common surgical problems.

Mr David Cade FRCS
Consultant General Surgeon
Associate Medical Director
Mid Cheshire Hospitals NHS Foundation Trust

Acknowledgements

I wish to acknowledge Mr David Corless (Upper GI), Mr Arif Khan and Mr CR Selvasekar (Colorectal), Mr Andrew Guy and Mr. Magdi Hanafy (General and Vascular), Mr SN Selvachandran (Breast), Mr John Slavin (Biliary and Pancreatic), Dr Maure O'Donoghue (Microbiology), Mr John Bache, (Accident and Emergency), Dr M Tee and Dr John Scally (Radiology) - all consultants from Mid Cheshire Hospitals NHS Foundation Trust and Mr Joe Phillip, Specialist Registrar in Urology. They have all seen the chapters relevant to their specialties and made very useful comments and suggestions. I thank Jonothan J Earnshaw, Consultant Vascular Surgeon, Gloucestershire Royal Hospital for his constructive suggestions and final editing of vascular chapters 23, 24 and 25.

Drs Padmasiri Perera (Psychiatry) and Suneetha Perera (Anaesthesia) made constructive comments that assisted the format of presentation.

I thank Professor Kumudu Wjewardene, Dean, Faculty of Graduate Studies and Senior Professor of Community Medicine, University of Sri Jayawardenepura, Sri Lanka, for critically reviewing several chapters.

The excellent support rendered by Nikki Bramhill (Director, tfm Publishing Ltd.) was an enormous strength to me. Her hard work, thirst for detail and focused professional approach decorated the book and made its completion in a record time a reality.

Finally, I would like to pay a very special tribute to Mr David Cade, Consultant Surgeon, Mid Cheshire Hospitals NHS Foundation Trust, for his guidance at all stages throughout the project. He read all the chapters and made very valuable comments and suggestions. As a respected trainer of surgeons with a wealth of experience in general surgery his enthusiastic support throughout has been invaluable to the success of the project.

Abbreviations

AAA Abdominal aortic aneurysm
ABPI Ankle brachial pressure index
ALP Alkaline phosphatase
ALT Alanine transaminase
APACHE Acute Physiology And Chronic Health Evaluation
APC Adenomatous polyposis coli
APR Abdominoperineal resection
APTT Activated partial thromboplastin time
ARDS Acute respiratory distress syndrome
AST Aspartate transaminase
ATLS® Advanced Trauma Life Support®
BASO British Association of Surgical Oncology
BD Twice a day
BMI Body mass index
BP Blood pressure
BPH Benign prostatic hypertrophy
BSG British Society of Gastroenterology
BUN Blood urea nitrogen
CBD Common bile duct
CCF Congestive cardiac failure
CEA Carcino-embryonic antigen
CLO Columnar-lined oesophagus
CNS Central nervous system
CO Carbon monoxide
COPD Chronic obstructive pulmonary disease
CRP C-reactive protein
CSF Cerebrospinal fluid
CT Computed tomography
CVP Central venous pressure
DCIS Ductal carcinoma *in situ*
DHT Dihydrotestosterone
DPL Diagnostic peritoneal lavage
DVT Deep vein thrombosis
ECG Electrocardiogram
EMR Endosocpic mucosal resection
ERCP Endoscopic retrograde cholangiopancreatography
ESR Erythrocyte sedimentation rate
ESWL Extracorporeal shock wave lithotripsy
EUA Examination under anaesthesia
EUS Endoscopic ultrasound
EVAR Endovascular aneurysm repair
FAP Familial adenomatous polyposis
FAST Focused assessment sonography for trauma
FBC Full blood count
Fe Iron
FMTC Familial medullary thyroid carcinoma
FNAC Fine needle aspiration cytology
FOB Faecal occult blood
GA General anaesthesia
GCS Glasgow Coma Scale
GGT Gamma glutamyl transpeptidase
GI Gastrointestinal
GORD Gastro-oesophageal reflux disease
GTN Glyceryl trinitrate
HCG Human chorionic gonadotrophin
Hb Haemoglobin
HDU High dependency unit
HNPCC Hereditary non-polyposis colorectal cancer
IBD Inflammatory bowel disease
IBS Irritable bowel syndrome
IC Indeterminate colitis
ICP Intracranial pressure
ICU Intensive care unit

IED Interstitial oedematous pancreatitis
IHD Ischaemic heart disease
IM Intestinal metaplasia
INR International Normalised Ratio
IPAA Ileal pouch anal anastomosis
I-PSS International Prostate Symptom Score
IVU Intravenous urogram
K Potassium
KUB Kidney, urethra, bladder
LCIS Lobular carcinoma *in situ*
LDH Lactate dehydrogenase
LMWH Low-molecular-weight heparin
LUTS Lower urinary tract symptoms
MDT Multidisciplinary team
MEN Multiple endocrine neoplasia
MRA Magnetic resonance angiography
MRCP Magnetic resonance cholangiopancreatogram
MRI Magnetic resonance imaging
MRSA Methicillin-resistant *Staphylococcus aureus*
MTC Medullary thyroid carcinoma
N Normal
Na Sodium
NG Nasogastric
NICE National Institute for Health and Clinical Excellence
NPI Nottingham Prognostic Index
NSAID Non-steroidal anti-inflammatory drug
PCNL Percutaneous nephrolithotomy
PE Pulmonary embolism
PET Positron emission tomography
PPI Proton pump inhibitor
PPPD Pylorus-preserving pancreatoduodenectomy
PSA Prostate specific antigen
PTBD Percutaneous transhepatic biliary drainage
PTH Parathyroid hormone
PTHrP Parathyroid hormone-related peptide
QOL Quality of life
RR Respiratory rate
S Serum
SIGN Scottish Intercollegiate Guidelines Network
TB Tuberculosis
TBSA Total body surface area
TCCP Tropical chronic calcific pancreatitis
TDLU Terminal duct lobular unit
TDS Three times a day
TIA Transient ischaemic attack
TIPS Transjugular intrahepatic portosytemic shunt
TLOSR Transient lower oesophageal sphincter relaxation
TME Total mesorectal excision
TSH Thyroid stimulating hormone
TURP Transurethral resection of the prostate
UC Ulcerative colitis
UTI Urinary tract infection
VTE Venous thromboembolism
WCC White cell count

Dedication

"This book is dedicated to all my teachers who gave of their time and made the effort to teach."

Chapter 1

The art of approaching a clinical problem

Learning objectives

- To recollect the clinical pathway to arrive at a diagnosis of common surgical presentations.

The transfer of textbook knowledge to a specific situation is a challenging task in clinical surgery. This process requires retention of information, the organisation and recall of facts, and the precise application to a given patient. Based on this recall, the clinician arrives at a clinical judgement on which he formulates a management plan.

The first step of this process is the gathering of information. This includes taking the patient's history, performing a physical examination, and obtaining laboratory results and results from other special examinations such as endoscopy. Of all, obtaining a good history is the most important and the most useful.

During the initial interview with the patient, it is good practice to allow and encourage the patient to explain the problem without interruptions. Some patients are excellent historians. However, some will have their own perceptions of the problem and at times this may mislead students and young doctors. Experienced clinicians use relevant or leading questions when the patient goes off at a tangent and also to fill the voids left in the patient's description. Selecting the relevant questions for a given clinical situation may pose a challenge to students and young doctors at an early stage of their training.

Presenting complaint

Recognition of the presenting complaint is an essential prerequisite to begin the process. A time tested technique is to begin by asking the main reason for seeking medical advice.

Duration of the presenting complaint

The duration of the presenting complaint is equally important because it may have a direct impact on the diagnosis. For example, abdominal pain which lasts for a few hours may be a biliary or renal colic, whereas chronic and periodic abdominal pain may be more suggestive of peptic ulceration.

History of the presenting complaint

The history of the presenting complaint helps the clinician to understand the background of the illness and to formulate a series of leading questions which will support or will help to exclude certain diagnoses. It is again good practice to enquire as to the precise time period commencing from a day or from a month when the patient was in normal health, and then to build a detailed history of the events or symptoms which the patient could recall 'from normal to abnormal'. Of course the case is expected to be built only upon the information obtained from the patient and the components cannot be added or ignored. The information obtained may not fit perfectly with the most likely diagnosis; this is not uncommon. The ability to recognise the most relevant information and to gather it accurately takes time and much practice.

The selection of leading questions pertinent to the case

At an early stage of training in surgery, students and young doctors are often incapable of recalling the relevant questions from their knowledge base when tested. This may be due to insufficient knowledge but, mostly, it is the inability to recognise the necessary information for a given clinical situation. Another tested technique for the early trainee in general surgery is, first to interview the patient, formulate the thought process on the evidence obtained and then to discuss the clinical scenario with one of the senior clinicians in the team managing the patient. This simple technique, if practised often, will help students and young doctors to recognise the deficient areas in their knowledge base. It will also help them to understand the reasons for not recognising the correct pathway to arrive at the most likely diagnosis and management plan. It is the technique and approach that students and young doctors must be eager to learn rather than simply attempting to memorise the factual knowledge of a clinical condition. The best way to master this art is by repeated practice and this is achieved by spending more time with patients on the surgical wards.

Organ/system diagnosis or recognition of the organ system

It is good practice to identify what is described as the organ/system diagnosis at the initial stage of history taking and then to think of a differential diagnosis. After a series of relevant or leading questions, the most likely diagnosis or the working diagnosis is reached. An experienced clinician may recognise the clinical problem with ease, which is a skill that is acquired with years of experience.

How the organ/system diagnosis, the most likely diagnosis and the working diagnosis are related in guiding clinical judgement is outlined below.

Organ diagnosis

Organ diagnosis will help to identify a series of relevant or leading questions related to the diseases or conditions which are specific to that organ system. The answers to these questions are the building blocks on which the case will be built.

A patient presenting with episodic loose stools, left-sided abdominal pain and a sense of incomplete evacuation of faeces is likely to have a disease in his colon or rectum.

Taking a patient with dysphagia as an example, the oesophagus will be the most likely organ and an obstructive lesion will be the most likely cause. But it is also possible that the stomach could be the likely organ and not the oesophagus. This is possible if the inlet of the stomach becomes obstructed due to gastric pathology.

Thinking of the possible causes of obstruction will bring further relevant questions to the mind. If the duration of dysphagia is long, for example, over 2 years, this information makes cancer less likely as the cause of the obstruction. Cancers can often progress rapidly and may not fit the overall appearance of the patient who may seem reasonably well. This will draw a list of further relevant questions for and against other benign disorders such as benign oesophageal strictures due to gastro-oesophageal reflux disease (GORD), corrosive strictures and achalasia of the cardia which can present with dysphagia. Has this patient had heartburn and acid regurgitation for a considerable length of time before the onset of dysphagia? If so, a benign oesophageal stricture due to longstanding reflux of hydrochloric acid should be considered because repeated reflux causes chronic oesophagitis which leads to fibrosis and stricture formation. Has he swallowed any corrosive substances in the past? If the answer is yes, then corrosive stricture as the cause of dysphagia is most likely, in which case the time of ingestion of the corrosive substance and the time of onset of the dysphagia become relevant to build the case further. Dysphagia for liquids and solids of longer duration will bring achalasia of the cardia into the picture. Considering the mechanism of achalasia, questions must be asked regarding the symptoms of nocturnal cough, that wake the patient when fluid refluxes into the larynx from the dilated oesophagus. Dilatation of the oesophagus in achalasia takes months or years to develop. Furthermore, if the patient admits passing fluid not only through the mouth but also through the nose during these nocturnal bouts of coughing, this is strong evidence of achalasia as the most likely cause of oesophageal obstruction. In the supine position when fluid in the dilated oesophagus fills the larynx, the patient will cough violently to avoid the acidic gastric juice from entering the trachea. Air pressure will then push the fluid from all possible openings including the nasal passages.

Cancer must also be considered as the most likely cause, especially if the dysphagia is of a short duration and is progressive. If the dysphagia is associated with a significant loss of appetite, carcinoma of the fundus of the stomach obstructing the gastric inlet should be considered because loss of appetite is one of the early symptoms seen in gastric cancer rather than in oesophageal cancer.

Some patients may volunteer additional information that at first glance may not appear relevant to the presenting problem. This type of information must be carefully scrutinised before being discarded.

The recognition of the involved organ system will facilitate the process of clinical decision making.

Most likely diagnosis

Working on a clinical case, it is not always possible at the end of history taking to make a definitive diagnosis. A list of differential diagnoses is considered, prioritised and the most likely diagnosis is first on the list. A comprehensive clinical examination including a digital examination of the natural orifices should then be performed. It is mandatory to have a chaperone present during clinical examination of female patients by a male doctor.

Investigations will help to set aside or support the most likely diagnosis. A management plan is then formulated.

Working diagnosis

A good example to understand how the working diagnosis applies to this process is to consider a clinical scenario of a middle-aged female with a palpable breast lump. This lump has no specific features that support any of the differential diagnoses such as cancer, fibroadenosis, a breast cyst or fibroadenoma. Therefore, after taking a history and conducting an examination, the surgeon may consider carcinoma of the breast as his working diagnosis until proven otherwise by histology. A working diagnosis is considered as an interim measure, particularly where missing a diagnosis such as cancer will have detrimental consequences for the patient.

Past medical and surgical history

Certain associated conditions may have an effect on the disease process or on the proposed treatment including surgery, and therefore need to be analysed carefully. For example, the control of diabetes becomes difficult in the presence of intra-abdominal suppuration until the pus is drained (continuing sepsis stimulates a stress reaction and the release of diabetogenic hormones). Also, some of the symptoms and signs may be due to comorbid conditions rather than the disease process itself. A patient with abdominal pain due to gallstones may also have bilateral ankle oedema due to congestive cardiac failure.

The past surgical history is important. A patient who has had abdominal surgery for cancer of the caecum in the past, presenting with the alteration of bowel habits may have developed another cancer in the colon; a metachronous cancer. A student or young doctor who has identified in a patient, who is awaiting surgery for gallstones, a past history of delayed recovery following surgery for an inguinal hernia under general anaesthesia due to suxamethonium apnoea (sux apnoea), will undoubtedly impress the surgical examiner!

A tendency towards depression and anxiety should be noted, as this may have an effect on the outcome of surgery.

Drug history and allergies

Many elderly patients are on multiple medications. Some drugs will have an effect on the symptoms and signs or may have a detrimental effect on the proposed surgery. Others may have to be discontinued prior to surgery. The doses may need to be altered to regulate the blood levels or they may have to be replaced with a substitute. For example, a patient who has intra-abdominal bleeding will not have tachycardia if he is on beta-blockers. Operating on a patient without recognising the fact that the patient is on warfarin is disastrous. A patient who is on long-term steroids undergoing surgery will need to be given a high dose of intravenous steroids to prevent an adrenal crisis.

It is important to enquire into the use of alternative medicines, especially from patients in the Asian subcontinent. Rarely some of these medications may contain significant quantities of alcohol and may be responsible for raised liver enzymes.

Allergies have to be asked about carefully in every surgical patient, as drugs may have to be given once the patient is anaesthetised and by then this cannot be verified from the patient. Latex allergy is becoming increasingly common in the modern world. Latex-free sets are available and in some institutions latex-free operating theatres are in use. Allergies to metals such as nickel have to be identified prior to laparoscopic surgery.

Social history

A detailed history of the quantity and duration of alcohol consumption, smoking and the possible use of illicit drugs should be obtained. Occupation, family background, family support that could be expected after surgery, and hobbies, may shed light on certain issues that may be relevant to the overall management of the patient.

Family history

A history of genetically transmitted disorders, a family history of cancer and the age of onset of such cancers should be noted. A family history of adverse reactions to anaesthetic medications, such as malignant hyperthermia, is significant because the condition has an autosomal dominant inheritance.

Systems review

A systems review should be performed with special emphasis on common diseases. In the elderly, symptoms suggestive of cardiac disease such as shortness of breath, chest pain or palpitations should be elicited. These findings will also be useful as a baseline for comparison during the postoperative period.

Physical examination

The golden rule of physical examination, inspection, palpation, percussion and auscultation cannot be over-emphasised. Summarised below is a general plan to be remembered:

- General appearance:
  - well nourished or cachetic;
  - calm or anxious.
- Vital signs:
  - pulse rate, heart rate, blood pressure, respiratory rate.
- Head and neck examination:
  - oral cavity, colour of the mucosa, lesions on the tongue and buccal mucosa;
  - lymph nodes;
  - other masses such as goitres;
  - oedema.
- Examination of breasts:
  - inspection. Symmetry, nipple and skin retraction (inspect with the patient's hands on their hips to contract the pectoralis muscle and then with the arms raised);
  - palpation. Masses, assessment of the nipples for discharges and palpation of the axillary, supraclavicular and abdominal lymph nodes and the liver.

- Abdominal examination:
  - inspection. Scars, distension, visible peristalsis, masses, skin discoloration (Grey Turner sign indicates retroperitoneal haemorrhage in acute pancreatitis);
  - palpation. Masses (retroperitoneal masses do not move with respiration), tenderness, guarding, rebound tenderness;
  - percussion. A dull note indicates solid masses or fluid; a resonant note means air; and a shifting dullness indicates ascites;
  - auscultation. Normal or high pitched bowel sounds.
- Examination of the respiratory system:
  - inspection. Respiratory rate and chest wall shape/movements (compare the two sides and look for paradoxical movement in a flail chest);
  - palpation. Chest wall movements, crepitus (surgical emphysema), local tenderness, deformity, abnormal mobility (sites of rib fractures); tracheal position (midline or deviated to one side, pushed away by fluid or by air, pulled towards by fibrosis or chronic collapse of the lung); and vocal fremitus (flat of the hand is kept on the affected part of the chest wall and the patient is asked to repeat a phrase such as 'ninety-nine'. A consolidated lung will transmit vibration when this is done);
  - percussion. Hyper-resonance in pneumothorax; stony dull in pleural effusion;
  - auscultation. Air entry (absent in pneumothorax and effusion, bronchial breathing in consolidation); vocal resonance (resonance of sounds in the chest made by the voice when the patient repeats a phrase, e.g. ninety-nine. A consolidated lung as in pneumonia conducts vibrations better than normal air-containing lung, so that the vocal resonance is increased); and added sounds (wheezes, crackles, pleural rub).
- Examination of the cardiovascular system:
  - pulse rate, rhythm and symmetry;
  - compare radial, brachial, carotid, femoral, popliteal and pedal pulses (a reduced or absent pulse indicates proximal obstruction to the arterial tree);
  - heart rate, rhythm, sounds, murmurs, clicks and rubs;
- Examination of the back and spine:
  - symmetry, swellings, movements, tenderness.
- Examination of the genitalia and groin:
  - males: scrotum for cystic and solid masses and the penis for phimosis, para-phimosis, hypospadias, growths and infections;
  - females: per-vaginal bimanual examination to elicit cervical tenderness, uterine and ovarian masses.

Clinical points

- The art of approaching a clinical problem:
  - recognise accurately the main reason(s) for seeking a medical consultation;
  - identify the most likely anatomical organ/system responsible for the clinical picture;
  - where necessary select leading questions considering the pathological conditions pertinent to the organ/system involved;
  - identify the pathological conditions that may be responsible and select the most likely condition;
  - remember common things are common and rare things are rare.

- Anal and rectal examination:
  - a direct inspection of the anus and assessment by gently separating the anal opening;
  - skin tags, external haemorrhoids, and limited view of internal haemorrhoids, fissures, peri-anal sinuses and suppurations;
  - digital examination;
  - prostate gland (enlargement, nodularity, tenderness, mobility of the mucosa, median groove);
  - other rectal masses;
  - blood and/or mucus on the examination finger.

Receiving information, organisation and recall of facts, and the precise application to a given patient in order to arrive at a clinical judgement, is an art which all students should master. Empathic communication during the initial interview will help to gain patient confidence.

Chapter 2

The art of solving a clinical problem

Learning objectives

- To learn the stepwise approach to solving common clinical problems.
- To appreciate the importance of repeated practice of recollection, analysis and the application of knowledge to clinical situations.

Clinicians follow a standard stepwise approach to solving clinical problems (Figure 1).

The **first step** is to arrive at a diagnosis or the most likely diagnosis.

The process is to recall information obtained during the history and examination and to place the key issues appropriately. For example, if abdominal pain after meals, periodicity, and the long-term use of non-steroidal anti-inflammatory agents are the key issues, peptic ulcer disease will head the list of differential diagnoses. Chronic intermittent abdominal pain radiating to the back, newly discovered diabetes and alcohol abuse will bring chronic pancreatitis to the head of the list. To prioritise further, experienced clinicans may direct leading questions by inquiring about pale frothy floating stools which cannot be flushed easily. Although chronic pancreatitis is the most likely diagnosis in this situation, investigations should be requested not only to confirm the diagnosis but also to exclude peptic ulcer disease and pancreatic cancer in the same patient.

The **second step** is to assess the severity or stage of the condition.

For example, if the clinical problem is haematemesis, the risk to the patient is based on the volume and rapidity of blood loss and this determines the management plan. In a patient with cancer, the stage of the cancer at the time of detection will direct the therapeutic approach.

Based on the stage and/or the severity of the condition, a treatment strategy that is perceived as the best approach is implemented. This is the **third step**.

The **fourth step** is to monitor the response to treatment.

The general condition of the patient and improvement of parameters such as pain or tenderness are subjective evidence of response. Investigations such as radiology, endoscopy or laboratory tests may be repeated and can be used as more objective evidence of the response to therapy. However, to a student or young doctor, this may be a challenging task because in many instances the patient's initial presentation may not provide a clear diagnosis. Therefore, to master the art of approaching and solving clinical problems, students and young doctors are advised to answer the following questions with each clinical problem. This approach will facilitate problem-based learning by enhancing the ability to

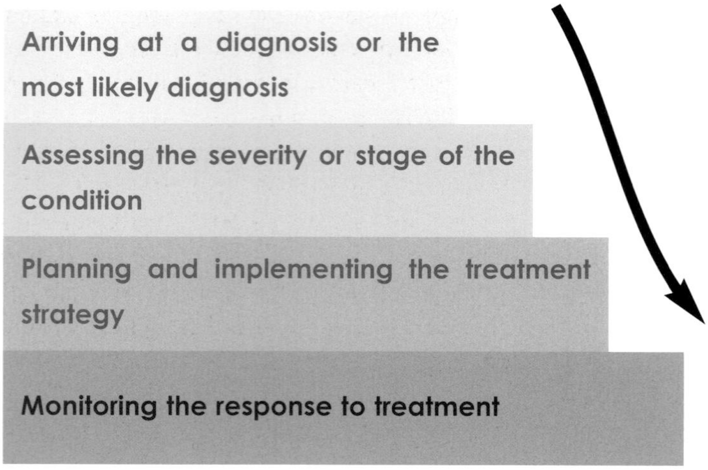

Figure 1. The stepwise approach to clinical problem solving.

acquire the essential core knowledge pertinent to the problem. More importantly it will help the learning process in applying the necessary components from the knowledge base to a given clinical situation:

- What is the most likely diagnosis?
- How do I justify my clinical judgement?
- How can I confirm the diagnosis?
- What should be my next step?
- What is the pathogenesis of this disease?
- What are the complications associated with this disease?
- What is the best treatment strategy for this patient?

Most of the questions are straightforward and the student should be able to come to a conclusion. A common stumbling block for many at an early stage of their training is: what should be my next step? This question is important and it may be a confusing issue for a student because that next step will often depend on the stage of solving the clinical problem. For example, the next step may be to obtain more information such as a histological confirmation or to decide the best of many treatment options. Students who learn and who are sometimes taught to regurgitate information about diseases may not be skilled enough to identify the next step. This is best learned at the bedside during case discussions with experienced clinical teachers who are prepared to listen and provide constructive feedback.

Given below are a few examples of well crafted assessments that could be expected from a good student or young doctor.

- At the stage of the diagnosis - the **next step**:

"I found a vague, slightly tender swelling in the right iliac fossa in Mr X who came in this morning with a clinical picture of intestinal obstruction. In view of his age, history of altered bowels, the 'feel' and tenderness of the swelling, I am concerned that he may be developing a closed loop obstruction with caecal distension. Therefore, I would request an urgent contrast CT scan of his abdomen to assess this situation."

- At the stage of assessing the severity of the condition - the **next step**:

"Mr X who had a laparotomy for peritonitis 8 months ago was admitted this morning with a 1-day history of abdominal pain. He has radiological evidence of small bowel obstruction which I think is most likely to be due to adhesions. Because he has no features suggestive of bowel ischaemia such as constant pain, fever, peritoneal signs or leucocytosis, my next step is to start him on a regime of nil by mouth, intravenous hydration, nasogastric aspiration and to keep him under constant review."

- Following the response to treatment - the **next step**:

"I need to assess Mr X who had a placement of a pancreatic stent after endoscopic sphincterotomy a month ago for chronic pancreatitis. I would like to study his pain scale chart to assess the feasibility of changing his medication from narcotic analgesics to a less strong analgesic."

What is the best therapy for this patient? is an important question to enable students and young doctors to learn the art of balancing the risks and benefits of a proposed intervention. For example, when managing a critically injured patient on the Advanced Trauma Life Support® (ATLS®) protocol, the best therapy will depend on (as highlighted in the case scenario in Chapter 16) the most likely immediate cause of death which is recognised during the primary survey. Immediate intubation is the best therapy for a road crash victim who has features of acute airway obstruction before a detailed assessment is conducted to rule out other injuries.

The repeated practice, focused reading to clarify facts and experience will make the art of problem solving an enjoyable exercise.

Chapter 3

Breast lump

Learning objectives

- To learn the initial work-up and staging of a patient with a newly diagnosed breast cancer.
- To understand the radiological, cytological and histopathological applications in breast cancer.
- To learn the basic pathology of breast cancer.
- To be familiar with the treatment options for locoregional and systemic disease and the basis for the selection of hormonal therapy.

Case scenario

A 60-year-old lady presents with a lump in her right breast. She found the lump 2 weeks ago whilst having a bath. She has two children that she breast fed and she has no family history of breast cancer.

On examination, both breasts are symmetrical and the nipples are not retracted. There is a 2.5cm x 2cm lump with ill-defined margins in the upper outer quadrant of the right breast. It is not attached to the deep structures but elevation of both arms shows slight puckering of the skin over the lump. There are no other skin changes and the axillary and supraclavicular lymph nodes are not palpable.

The chest and abdominal examinations are normal.

The most likely clinical diagnosis: carcinoma of the right breast.

Clinical points

- Puckering of the skin strongly indicates that there is an underlying malignant lesion. This physical sign is highly suggestive of cancer.

The maximum diameter of the tumour is 2.5cm. Therefore, this is a T2 tumour according to the TNM classification. Clinical TNM staging of this patient is T2 N0 Mx (Table 1).

What is the TNM classification? (T - tumour, N - nodes, M - metastases)

The TNM classification (Table 1) is a clinical assessment which takes into account the tumour size, the lymph node status and the presence of metastases. This staging is important because the prognosis of the cancer relates to the stage at presentation. However, because the TNM classification depends on the clinical measurement of tumour size and the lymph node status, both of these are not accurate pre-operatively. To improve the system, the tumour size and lymph node status are assessed by the pathologist after surgery.

What is the next step?

- The patient should have a triple assessment:
  - clinical examination - already done;
  - mammogram and ultrasound imaging;
  - needle biopsy/tissue sampling (fine needle aspiration cytology [FNAC] or core biopsy).

What is a mammogram?

A mammogram is an X-ray of the breast tissue (Figures 1 and 2). When a small dose of ionising radiation passes through human tissue, depending on the amount of radiation absorbed, it will appear different in the film. The fatty tissue which surrounds the glandular breast tissue absorbs the least amount of radiation. As young women have dense glandular breast tissue, mammograms may not be very helpful because they cannot differentiate between tumour tissue which is usually dense from the dense glandular tissue. Therefore, mammograms are of less value in women under 35, and mammograms are not usually

Table 1. TNM classification.

- T - tumour.
- N - nodes.
- M - metastases.

The tumour measurement is made on physical examination.

Primary tumour (T):
- T1: tumour not larger than 2.0cm in the greatest dimension.
- T2: tumour larger than 2.0cm but not larger than 5.0cm in the greatest dimension.
- T3: tumour larger than 5.0cm in the greatest dimension.
- T4: tumour of any size with direct extension to the chest wall or to the skin.

Skin involvement means either:
- Oedema (including peau d'orange).
- Ulceration of the skin of the breast over the lump.
- Satellite skin nodules confined to the same breast.

Regional lymph nodes (N):
- N0: no palpable regional lymph nodes.
- N1: palpable mobile ipsilateral axillary lymph nodes.
- N2: palpable fixed ipsilateral axillary lymph nodes.

Distant metastases (M):
- M0: no distant metastases.
- M1: distant metastases are present. This includes ipsilateral supraclavicular nodes.
- Mx: distant metastases, not assessed

done, although they can be ordered if there is a suspicion on clinical examination, cytology or biopsy that the patient may have cancer.

In older women, the functional glandular tissue diminishes leaving only thin supporting tissues clearly outlined by the fatty tissue. Mammograms in these 'mature' breasts are very effective, since even small cancers are well outlined by the fat. In addition, breast cancers may develop calcium deposits which are easily seen on a mammogram. These are called microcalcifications.

However, microcalcifications of the breast are very common, and are seen in about 86% of mammograms. They are usually benign calcifications in the ducts, the frequency of which increases with age. Benign calcifications are usually larger then calcifications associated with malignancy. They are coarser and often round with smooth margins. The calcifications associated with breast cancer are usually very small and often the use of a magnifying glass is necessary to see them. Certain morphological characteristics such as branching and casting are highly suspicious of malignancy.

In order to standardise mammography reporting, the American College of Radiology has implemented the Breast Imaging Reporting And Database System, known as BIRADS. In addition to the morphological features, the BIRADS takes into account other well established attributes such as shape, size, density, number, distribution, location and associated findings.

Clinical points

- Because breasts are relatively radiodense in women aged under 35, mammography is rarely of value below this age.

What is the difference between a plain X-ray and a mammogram?

Mammograms are performed by special machines which compress the breast between two plates (Figure 1). The compression evens out the breast thickness so that all the tissues can be seen and because the tissue is spread out, small abnormalities will not be obscured by the overlying breast tissue.

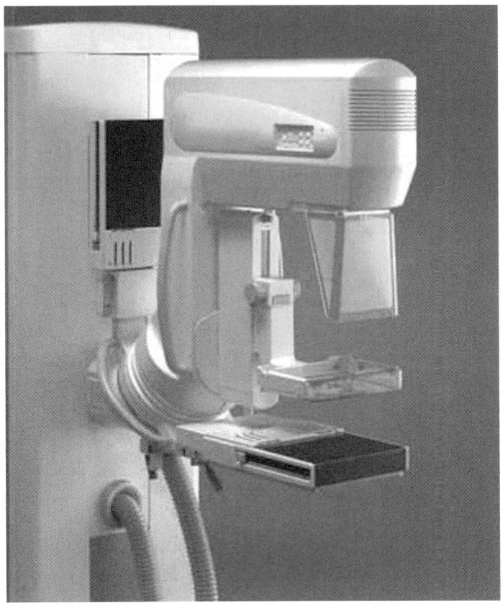

Figure 1. Mammography machine.

Mass lesions and areas of parenchymal distortion are also suspicious of cancer and can be detected by mammography. In mammography:

- Cysts are shown as transparent objects.
- Benign solid lesions have well demarcated edges.
- Cancers usually have an indistinct margin.

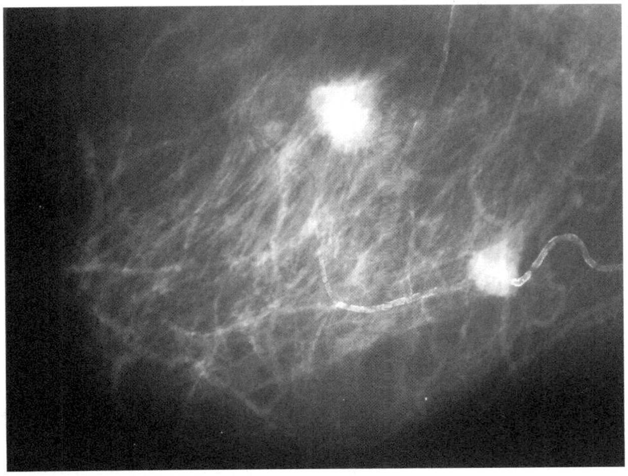

Figure 2. Mammogram of a multifocal breast cancer, showing two lesions and microcalcification. ***Reproduced with permission from Mr SN Selvachandran, Consultant Breast Surgeon, Leighton Hospital, Crewe, UK.***

What is the role of breast ultrasound?

Breast ultrasound is very useful when evaluating a breast lump because it can differentiate between cystic and solid tissue. It is a valuable assessment tool in women of any age and in particular below 35, where mammography is of limited value. Ultrasound is not, however, a screening investigation, and is of no value in the normal breast.

Progress of the patient

- The mammogram shows an area of parenchymal deformity with indistinct margins corresponding to the palpable lump in the upper outer quadrant of the right breast. Another suspicious mass is also seen in the upper medial quadrant of the same breast. This lesion is not palpable. No enlarged lymph nodes can be felt in the axilla.
- The ultrasound confirms that the palpable lump is solid.

What is the next step?

- To obtain a tissue diagnosis of both lesions.
- Ultrasound-guided core biopsies of both lesions are performed.

What is a core biopsy?

A small core of tissue is removed from the lump or from the suspected area under ultrasound guidance using a cutting needle. This is a special needle which cuts into and delivers the cut tissue with the needle. Several cores or pieces are removed for histology.

Why is fine needle aspiration cytology (FNAC) not considered in this patient?

This would have been the obvious alternative. In FNAC, the cells are sucked out from the lesion using a needle and syringe for cytological analysis. A sufficient quantity of cells and the expertise of a pathologist are needed for accurate interpretation. Although it has a high sensitivity, it also has a small percentage of false positives. The core biopsy, if correctly performed from the site, has an almost zero false positive rate. Therefore, if the expertise is available to perform core biopsies, a tissue diagnosis is better than a cytological diagnosis.

Core biopsies will also differentiate an invasive carcinoma from an *in situ* carcinoma. This information is relevant to the future management.

How does a pathologist report on FNAC?

C indicates that the reporting is on cells and not on a tissue sample:

- C1 - inadequate sample.
- C2 - benign.
- C3 - atypical cells - probably benign.
- C4 - suspicious of malignancy.
- C5 - malignant.

For core biopsies, B indicates that it is a biopsy:

- B1 - unsatisfactory or normal tissue only.
- B2 - benign.
- B3 - uncertain malignant potential.
- B4 - suspicious of malignancy.
- B5a - *in situ* malignancy.
- B5b - invasive malignancy.

Progress of the patient

- The core biopsy of the palpable mass is reported as an invasive ductal carcinoma (B5b).
- The tissue obtained from the lesion in the upper medial quadrant of the same breast is reported as a ductal carcinoma *in situ* (DCIS) (B5a).

What is the difference between an *in situ* carcinoma and an infiltrative carcinoma?

The functional unit of the breast is the terminal duct lobular unit (TDLU) which consists of lobules and terminal ducts that drain milk via the duct system to the nipple. The cells of the TDLU undergo changes that develop benign, pre-cancerous and cancerous breast disease. Therefore, the cells of origin of a breast cancer lie within the TDLU. Most breast cancers are ductal cancers.

Tumours that arise from the cells that line the breast ducts are called duct carcinomas and those that arise from lobules are called lobular carcinomas. At an early stage the cancer cells of either type are confined to the basement membrane and are referred to as carcinoma *in situ*, e.g. DCIS (ductal carcinoma *in situ*) or LCIS (lobular carcinoma *in situ*). When the tumour breaks through the basement membrane to the surrounding breast tissue, it becomes an invasive cancer. This is a histological distinction (and cannot be made on cytology).

Some breast cancers show distinct patterns of growth and cellular morphology. On this basis certain special types of breast cancer can also be identified (tubular, mucoid, papillary or cribriform). This has some clinical relevance because some of these special types have a better prognosis. For example, the papillary type of breast cancer has a better prognosis than other types.

What is the next step?

- The case is discussed at the multidisciplinary team (MDT) meeting.

What is a multidisciplinary team?

It is now widely accepted that multidisciplinary teams (MDT) form the basis for best practice in the management of breast cancer. These teams usually consist of breast surgeons, medical oncologists with a special interest in breast cancer, pathologists, radiologists, breast care nurses and data management personnel. The team meets regularly to discuss the best management plan for each patient.

Progress of the patient

- The case is discussed and the decision is made to advise a mastectomy as the best option for the two breast lesions. Breast conservation surgery is not considered as an option because this patient has multifocal disease in the right breast.

What is breast conservation surgery?

Three surgical options are available for the local control of breast cancer. These are:

- Mastectomy (removal of the whole breast).
- Wide local excision (excision of the tumour with a 1cm resection margin).
- More extensive excision of a whole quadrant of the breast (quadrantectomy).

The latter two options are referred to as breast conservation surgery.

Clinical points

- This patient has multifocal disease in her right breast and therefore she cannot be considered for breast conservation surgery.

Mastectomy is an extremely sensitive issue for women. Patients should be actively involved in decision making about their surgical treatment. A safe choice is not always possible and patients need to know the advantages and disadvantages of a particular course of action. Involvement of specialist breast care nurses at this stage can be very helpful.

Patients who undergo breast conservation therapy are usually offered radiotherapy to the affected breast. Postoperative radiotherapy has been shown to reduce the long-term risk of local recurrence following breast conservation surgery.

Major randomised trials comparing breast conservation surgery with radiotherapy versus mastectomy for invasive breast cancer have shown that the risk of local recurrence after breast conservation surgery and radiotherapy is 1.5 to 2 times greater than following mastectomy, and further surgery may become necessary. However, there is no evidence that the long-term prognosis is worse after wide local excision and radiotherapy, provided the guidelines on treatment are followed, especially as regards to completeness of the excision.

The British Association of Surgical Oncology (BASO) guidelines suggest that the units performing breast surgery should achieve a local recurrence rate after breast conservation of less than 10% with a target of 5%.

Clinical points

- Patients after breast conservation surgery are usually treated with radiotherapy to the affected breast.
- The risk of local recurrence following breast conservation surgery is 1.5 to 2 times higher than after mastectomy but there is no evidence that survival is adversely affected.
- Completeness of the excision, lymphatic or vascular invasion, an extensive *in situ* component, histological grade and the age of the patient are recognised factors associated with the risk of local recurrence.

What are the criteria for breast conservation therapy?

Small non-centrally placed tumours

The single most important factor that influences local recurrence after breast conservation surgery is the completeness of the excision with adequate margins. Therefore, most breast units will consider tumours of 4cm or less for breast conservation. Adequate excision of lesions above 4cm may well cause poor cosmetic results. Central lesions may produce unacceptable cosmetic results since the nipple may need to be removed, but the location in itself is not a major factor if the lesion is small.

If the patient has a tumour which is too large to achieve a satisfactory cosmetic result then initial treatment with systemic chemotherapy (neoadjuvant treatment) might well shrink the tumour sufficiently to allow a satisfactory result from conservative surgery at a later date, without compromising long-term survival. Alternatively, the patient can be offered mastectomy and primary breast reconstruction at the same operation.

Lower grade tumours

This is a histological grading based on the degree of differentiation of the tumour cells. This grading is known as the Bloom and Richardson grade. It provides good prognostic information for both the disease-free interval and overall survival.

Three groups, grade 1 to 3, are identified. Grade 1 is shown to have a lower recurrence rate by a factor of 1.5 compared with grades 2 and 3.

Absence of lymphatic or vascular invasion

Lymphatic or vascular invasion are both markers of aggressive disease. These tumours are at increased risk of local and systemic recurrence.

What is the best management of the axilla?

The presence or absence of axillary lymph node involvement is the single best predictor of survival after breast cancer and management decisions are based on this. It is therefore important to have an accurate assessment of the axillary node status of this patient.

The patient has no clinically palpable axillary lymph nodes. The mammogram and ultrasound scan have not detected axillary lymph nodes. However, clinical examination and imaging are not sufficiently reliable indicators to predict the involvement of axillary nodes. Only 70% of involved axillary lymph nodes are clinically palpable. Involvement of axillary lymph nodes occurs in up to 50% of symptomatic breast cancers and 10-20% of screen-detected breast cancers.

Clinical points

- The presence or absence of axillary lymph node involvement is the single best predictor for survival in patients with breast cancer.

What pre-operative investigations are needed to rule out metastatic disease in this patient?

All patients should have a full blood count (FBC), chest X-ray and liver function tests to rule out any gross evidence of metastatic disease.

According to BASO guidelines, patients with a 'tumour only' or 'tumour with palpable nodes' need not have a bone scan and liver ultrasound/CT to search for occult metastases, unless the patient has specific symptoms or signs, or has an abnormal liver profile.

What is the next step?

- This patient needs a tissue diagnosis of the axillary node status. The patient is given three options (she is informed that any of these options can be performed concurrently with the mastectomy):
  - axillary clearance;
  - axillary node sampling;
  - sentinel lymph node biopsy.

What is axillary clearance?

The axillary lymph nodes receive about 95% of the lymph drainage of the breast. On average, there are about 20 lymph nodes in the axilla. They are divided into three groups in anatomical relation to the pectoralis minor muscle. Level I are the nodes which are situated lateral to the muscle, level II are the nodes found under the origin of the muscle and level III nodes are those found between the medial border of the pectoralis minor, first rib and the axillary vein, high in the axilla. Therefore, mastectomy and level II or III axillary node clearance can be offered to this patient at the same time through the same incision. There is evidence that axillary clearance offers the best control of axillary disease; however, it can produce long-term complications such as pain and lymphoedema.

What is axillary node sampling?

Dissecting out a minimum of four separate nodes is considered to be representative of all axillary nodes. The probability of false negatives decreases with the increasing number of harvested nodes.

What is sentinel node biopsy?

The first lymph node draining the site of a cancer is known as the sentinel node. This can be identified by injecting a blue dye and/or a radio-isotope colloid around the site of the tumour (peritumoural injection) and dissecting the axilla to harvest the node(s) stained blue or found to contain radio-isotope. More than one node is often identified. These nodes are assessed histologically.

If the sentinel node is negative, no further local treatment to the axilla is required If it is positive, the patient is given a choice between axillary radiotherapy or axillary clearance.

Two large randomised trials have found that sentinel node biopsy is an accurate diagnostic tool in patients with clinically node-negative breast cancer. This management approach has shown considerable improvement in morbidity rates when compared with standard axillary surgery.

Clinical points

- The first lymph node draining the site of a cancer is known as the sentinel node.
- If the sentinel node is negative, no further local treatment to the axilla is required.
- If positive, the patient is given a choice between axillary radiotherapy or axillary node clearance.
- Sentinel node biopsy is an accurate diagnostic tool in patients with clinically node-negative breast cancer.

Progress of the patient

- The patient selects sentinel node biopsy which is performed at the time of the mastectomy. This is reported as positive.
- At the next MDT meeting further management of the patient is discussed.
- The pathology report of the mastectomy specimen confirms the same findings as the core biopsy report:
  - palpable lump - infiltrative duct carcinoma;
  - impalpable lesion - DCIS.
- Tumour grade - Bloom and Richardson grade II.
- Tumour receptor status - oestrogen and progesterone receptor positive (ER+, PR+; ER = oestrogen receptors, PR = progesterone receptors).
- Nottingham Prognostic Index - 4.5 (see later).
- Options for the axilla are radiotherapy or axillary clearance.
- At the next clinic visit, soon after the results are available, the medical oncologist accompanied by the specialist breast nurse, discuss the results of histology and the treatment choices for the axillary disease with the patient.

Progress of the patient

- The patient selects axillary radiotherapy. Because she has an ER-positive tumour and she is postmenopausal, she is commenced on an aromatase inhibitor (anastrozole 1mg/day orally). Calcium 500mg and vitamin D 400 IU are added, since long-term treatment with aromatase inhibitors is known to be associated with an increased risk of osteoporosis.

What is the Nottingham Prognostic Index (NPI)?

Although individual factors are useful to predict prognosis, combining the independent variables in the form of an index allows identification of groups of patients with different prognoses. The Nottingham Prognostic Index is the most widely used and incorporates three prognostic factors: tumour size, node status and histological grade:

NPI = (0.2 X size) + node stage + grade.

Thus, the patient's NPI is:

NPI = (0.2 X 2.5cm) + 2 + 2 = 4.5.

Node stage:
1 = no nodes.
2 = 1-3.
3 = 4 or more.

What are aromatase inhibitors?

To understand the role of aromatase inhibitors it is first necessary to understand the role of oestrogens in breast cancer.

The natural history of breast cancer is closely linked with oestrogens. Tumours which are oestrogen positive have oestrogen receptors on the surface of the tumour cells. Oestrogen attaches to these receptor sites and 'switches on' the cancer cells to grow. Before the menopause, oestrogen is produced by the ovaries. Therefore, in a premenopausal patient the continuous stimulus by oestrogens can be stopped, either by blocking the receptor sites or by removing the source of oestrogen production.

In a premenopausal patient, the source of oestrogen production can be eliminated by open surgical or laparoscopic removal of the ovaries, or by irradiating them. More often, the receptor sites can be blocked by a drug called tamoxifen which is a synthetic molecule similar to the structure of the oestrogen molecule. Tamoxifen competes with oestrogen for the receptor sites on the surface of the cancer cells but unlike oestrogen, the tamoxifen molecule will not 'switch on' the cells. As the receptor sites are blocked by tamoxifen, oestrogen cannot stimulate the cells to grow. Women with ER-negative tumours derive no benefit from tamoxifen treatment.

After the menopause, the ovaries cease to function. But in the postmenopausal patient, oestrogen is still produced. This is by the conversion of androgens from the adrenal glands to oestrogens. Oestrogen production in the postmenopausal patient takes place in the adipose tissue, muscle and in the breast. An enzyme called aromatase is responsible for the last step of the process of conversion of androgens to oestrogens and the aromatase inhibitors block this step. As oestrogen in premenopausal patients are produced by the ovaries, there is no place for aromatase inhibitors in premenopausal patients.

Why is tamoxifen not considered in this patient?

This would have been an alternative. In fact, many postmenopausal patients are given tamoxifen therapy. The drug has a good safety record but there is a slightly increased risk of uterine cancer and deep venous thrombosis with long-term tamoxifen therapy. Several recent trials have confirmed that the disease-free interval is significantly longer and the distant recurrence rates are significantly lower in patients who are on aromatase inhibitors, compared with patients on tamoxifen, hence the reason for commencing aromatase inhibitors in this patient.

If this patient had been premenopausal, would there be a difference in management?

Yes. This patient has multifocal breast cancer with axillary disease. She is a candidate for adjuvant treatment with chemotherapy, especially if her tumour was ER-negative. The term 'adjuvant therapy' is used to describe chemotherapy, hormone therapy or radiotherapy given after surgery.

In general adjuvant chemotherapy is considered for almost all premenopausal patients with high grade invasive cancers, even in patients who are ER-positive.

What is neoadjuvant treatment?

Specific cancer treatment given before surgery is called neoadjuvant therapy. This may be hormonal treatment, such as an aromatase inhibitor, radiotherapy or chemotherapy. The main objective is to downstage or shrink the tumour prior to surgery. It may also provide an early indication of the expected response to a specific chemotherapy regime.

Progress of the patient

- The patient has an uneventful postoperative period and tolerates radiotherapy well. She is on long-term aromatase inhibitors and is currently under follow-up.

Suggested reading

1. American College of Radiology (ACR). Breast Imaging Reporting And Data System atlas (BI-RADS[R] atlas). Reston, VA: American College of Radiology, 2003.
2. The Association of Breast Surgery @ BASO; Royal College of Surgeons of England. Guidelines for the management of symptomatic breast disease. *Eur J Surg Oncol* 2005; 31: S1-21.
3. Blamey RW. The design and clinical use of Nottingham Prognostic Index in breast cancer. *Breast* 1996; 5: 156-7.
4. Noguchi M. Avoidance of axillary lymph node dissection in selected patients with node-positive breast cancer. *Eur J Surg Oncol* 2008; 34: 129-34.

Self-assessment

Q1
EMQ

a. Right mastectomy and axillary clearance.
b. Wide local excision, sentinel node sampling, and tamoxifen therapy.
c. Radiotherapy to the right breast and tamoxifen therapy.
d. Right mastectomy and sentinel node biopsy.
e. Radiotherapy to the right breast.

Select the most appropriate next step from the options given above for the case scenarios described below.

1. A 60-year-old lady presents with a 2.5cm x 2cm lump in the right breast. A mammogram reveals an area of microcalcification corresponding to the palpable lump. Another suspicious mass which is clinically impalpable is seen in the upper medial quadrant of the same breast. The core biopsy of the palpable lump identifies an ER-positive, invasive ductal carcinoma and the impalpable lesion is a ductal carcinoma *in situ*.
2. A 70-year-old lady presents with a 2.5cm x 2cm lump in the upper outer quadrant of the right breast. A mammogram reveals an area of microcalcification corresponding to the palpable lump. The core biopsy identifies an ER-positive, invasive ductal carcinoma.

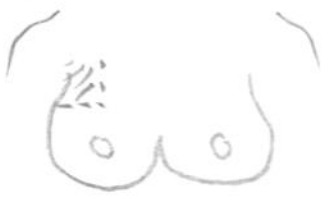

3. A sentinel node biopsy performed during a wide local excision with clear margins of an ER-positive, PR-positive, infiltrating right breast carcinoma in a 70-year-old lady is reported as negative.

Q2
SBA

A 65-year-old woman has breast conservation surgery for a 1.5cm-diameter, ER-negative, well differentiated duct carcinoma of the right breast with sentinel node sampling. Her sentinel node is negative for cancer.

What is the most appropriate next step in the management of this patient?

a. A course of chemotherapy.
b. Mastectomy and axillary clearance.
c. Radiation therapy to the affected breast.
d. No further treatment and routine follow-up.
e. Commence on tamoxifen.

Q3
True/False

The sentinel axillary lymph node:

a. Is the first node in the group of lymph nodes that drains the site of a cancer.
b. Is the node that contains cancer metastases.
c. Is the node which is at the apex of the axilla.
d. Is the node found closest to the lateral resection margin of the tumour.
e. If negative for cancer cells, no further local treatment to the axilla is required.

Q4
True/False

a. TNM staging of a 2.5cm-diameter tumour in the left breast with skin ulceration over its surface and a palpable mobile left lymph node is T2 N1 Mx.
b. The presence of microcalcification of branching type on mammography is suspicious of breast cancer.
c. All patients who undergo breast conservation surgery are advised to undergo local radiotherapy to the same breast.
d. The presence or absence of axillary lymph node involvement is the single best predictor of survival in breast cancer.
e. Aromatase inhibitors have no role in the treatment of breast cancer in premenopausal patients.

Q5
True/False

a. The incidence of breast cancer increases with age.
b. Nulliparity increases the life-time risk of breast cancer.
c. BRCA1 and BRCA2 are recognised breast cancer genes.
d. Breast cancer discovered during the second trimester of pregnancy should be treated by mastectomy and axillary clearance.
e. Klinefelter's syndrome is a risk factor for breast cancer in men.

Q6
True/False

The following are true/false of nipple discharge in women:

a. The majority are due to benign conditions.
b. The commonest cause of blood-stained nipple discharge is a duct papilloma.
c. Galactorrhoea is associated with the use of psychotrophic drugs.
d. Galactorrhoea is a manifestation of a pituitary tumour.
e. All patients with nipple discharge above the age of 40 should have mammography.

Answers overleaf

Self-assessment answers

Q1 1. (d), 2. (b), 3. (c).

Explanatory notes

1. This patient has a multifocal breast carcinoma with positive axillary nodes. Therefore, breast conservation would not be considered because of the increased risk of local recurrence with breast conservation. Mastectomy is the most appropriate option for her breast lesion. The axillary disease needs to be assessed with a sentinel node biopsy.

2. This patient has a localised T2 lesion in the upper outer quadrant of her right breast. Breast conservation can be considered. Wide local excision is recommended for a T2 lesion and she will need radiotherapy to the affected breast. The results of sentinel node biopsy will determine the treatment for the axilla.

3. This postmenopausal patient has a localised T2 lesion with a node-negative axilla. All she needs is adjuvant breast radiotherapy to reduce the risk of local recurrence.

Q2 (c).

Q3 a. (T), b. (F), c. (F), d. (F), e. (T).

Q4 a. (F), b. (T), c. (T), d. (T), e. (T).

Q5 a. (T), b. (T), c. (T), d. (T), e. (T).

Q6 a. (T), b. (T), c. (T), d. (T), e. (T).

Chapter 4

Biliary colic

Learning objectives

- To learn the varying clinical presentations of patients with symptomatic gallstone disease.
- To recollect the pathogenesis of gallstone disease.
- To learn the process of clinical judgement and decision making to arrive at the best treatment option for a patient with acute cholecystitis.

Case scenario

A 50-year-old obese woman presents with abdominal pain. The pain commenced about 2 hours after dinner. It was a dull ache which began in the epigastric region but with time it increased in severity and radiated to the right hypochondrium. The pain was so intense that she had to come to the hospital at midnight. She has no past history of dyspeptic symptoms or any other significant comorbid conditions.

On examination she looks unwell and has a temperature of 38.4°C. Her other vital signs are normal. The abdominal examination reveals mild right hypochondrial tenderness but no other abnormal physical signs.

She is given 50mg of pethidine intravenously to which she responds. The pain disappears when she wakes up in the morning but a dull ache in the right hypochondrium is persisting.

The results of her investigations are:

- White cell count (WCC) - 14,000/mm^3.
- Liver profile - normal.
- Serum (S) amylase - normal.
- The ultrasound scan shows multiple gallbladder stones, a thick-walled gallbladder and a normal common bile duct with a diameter of 5mm.

The most likely clinical diagnosis: biliary colic leading to early acute cholecystitis.

It is important to recognise the pathological process involving the extrahepatic biliary tree to formulate the best treatment strategy (Figure 1). The site, the severity and the radiation of pain in this patient is compatible with a clinical diagnosis of biliary colic. This is further supported by the fact that the pain has subsided almost completely by the morning, indicating that the stone which blocked the outlet of the gallbladder may have fallen back to the gallbladder or passed through to the bile duct.

However, the high white cell count (WCC), the tenderness in the right hypochondrium and the sonographic evidence of a thick-walled gallbladder with stones is indicative of an acute inflammatory process leading to oedema of the gallbladder wall; hence, the diagnosis of acute cholecystitis.

Could this picture be due to acute on chronic cholecystitis?

It is possible but is not the most likely diagnosis. Chronic cholecystitis results when the wall of the gallbladder reacts to the prolonged presence of gallstones in the gallbladder. These patients have significant dysfunction of the gallbladder. They present with dyspepsia, right hypochondrial discomfort and/or pain, and fat intolerance. The typical patient is often described as a fat, forty, flatulent, fertile female with the above mentioned symptoms. Of course many patients with gallstones do not fit this description. When acute inflammation develops on a background of chronic cholecystitis, the patient may present with an acute episode.

Acute on chronic cholecystitis is unlikely as this patient has no past history suggestive of dyspepsia and this is her first presentation. As such, the most likely diagnosis is biliary colic leading to early acute cholecystitis.

This patient has had severe epigastric pain and pyrexia. Could this be due to acute cholangitis?

Severe epigastric pain and pyrexia may represent acute cholangitis in patients with gallbladder stones. This is because it is possible that a stone may pass into the bile duct and during its attempted passage to the duodenum, it may become stranded at the sphincter of Oddi at the lower end of the bile duct. The resultant biliary stasis soon becomes infected causing acute cholangitis. Acute pyogenic cholangitis is a surgical emergency which has to be recognised early.

Bile duct obstruction with sepsis is invariably associated with at least some of the other features of extrahepatic ductal obstruction such as jaundice, pale stools, dark urine and pruritus. These patients also have biochemical evidence of hepatic dysfunction with elevation of all liver enzymes.

In the absence of the above features, it is unlikely that this patient has acute cholangitis.

Could she have empyema of the gallbladder?

If her condition is not recognised and treated early she may well develop empyema as a sequel to acute cholecystitis. Empyema is a collection of pus in the gallbladder, if the stage of acute inflammation advances to the stage of suppuration. This may happen if the stone continues to obstruct the gallbladder outlet and the condition is not recognised and treated with antibiotics. Her pain commenced after dinner, she presented to the hospital that night and the pain had subsided by the morning. She is pyrexial and has a raised white cell count. The duration of this scenario is not sufficient for her to have developed suppuration. She is not a diabetic, is not on steroids and has no immune deficiency or any other significant comorbid factors. One would have expected to observe a more poorly patient if she had pus in the gallbladder. Her abdominal findings are also not compatible with empyema. An inflamed gallbladder filled with pus is usually associated with significant pericholecystitis which means that there is some fluid around the inflamed gallbladder. The inflamed gallbladder irritates the parietal peritoneum and causes constant right hypochondrial pain, tenderness, guarding, rebound tenderness and some rigidity. However, the typical physical signs may not be elicited because of the obesity.

Acute empyema may lead to necrosis, gangrene, perforation and peritonitis. But this patient has no such picture.

Is her clinical picture compatible with acute gallstone pancreatitis?

It is possible as we are seeing the patient within the first 24 hours. She may well have passed a stone to the bile duct and from there during its passage through the ampulla of Vater, the stone may transiently obstruct the common channel and cause acute gallstone pancreatitis. The clinical picture within the first 24 hours is not incompatible with acute pancreatitis although she has no back pain.

A fact pointing against this diagnosis is that her serum amylase is normal. This would not exclude early acute pancreatitis because in about 10% of patients, the serum amylase may be normal in the early stages.

If the patient's condition deteriorates the serum amylase should be repeated and the serum lipase should be estimated. A raised serum lipase is a reliable indicator of acute pancreatitis.

Could this clinical picture be due to a mucocele of the gallbladder?

It is very unlikely. The classic picture of a mucocele occurs in a patient who has had a recent episode of biliary colic who presents with a palpable lump in the right hypochondrium.

The ultrasound scan will confirm a markedly distended gallbladder but no other evidence of extrahepatic ductal obstruction. The pathogenesis is believed to be an obstruction to the cystic duct when the gallbladder is relatively empty of bile. Mucous glands in the gallbladder wall secrete abnormal quantities of mucus which fills the gallbladder. There is no significant infection. The clinical picture of this patient is not compatible with this process.

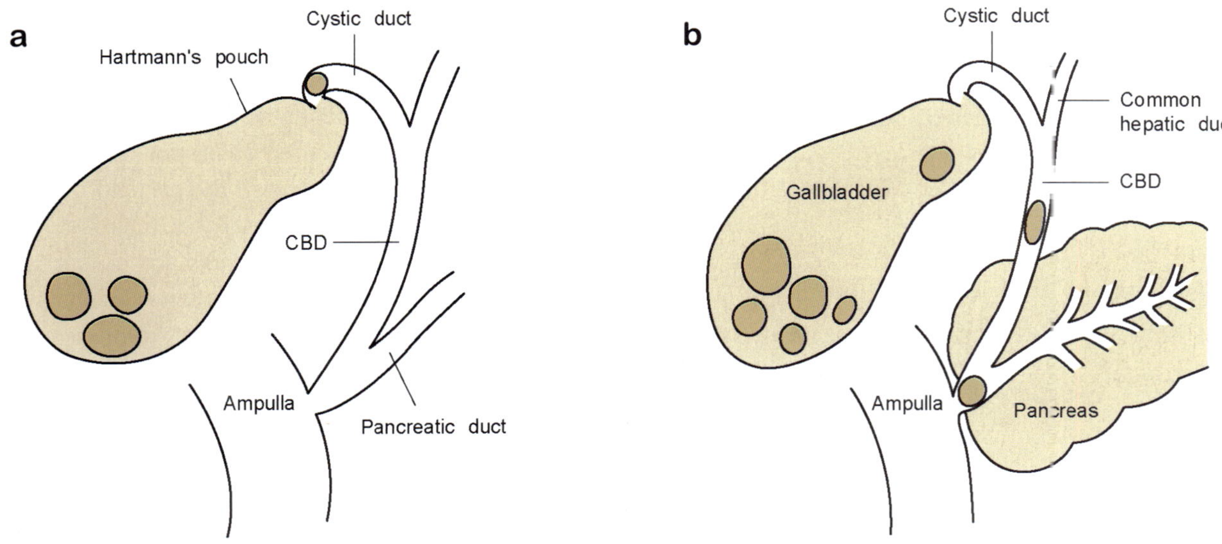

Figure 1. A graphic illustration of the pathogenesis of symptomatic gallstone disease.

Table 1. Complications of gallstones.

Gallbladder stones

- Acute cholecystitis.
- Empyema.
- Perforation.
- Chronic cholecystitis.
- Mucocele.

Bile duct stones

- Acute cholangitis.
- Obstructive jaundice.
- Acute pancreatitis.

What is the next step?

- Nil by mouth.
- Intravenous fluids.
- Intravenous antibiotics:
  - broad-spectrum antibiotics such as a second generation cephalosporin (cefuroxime 750mg IV stat and 750mg IV 8-hourly or ciprofloxacin 500mg IV b.d.).
- Deep vein thrombosis (DVT) prophylaxis:
  - low-molecular-weight heparin subcutaneously;
  - obesity and lack of mobility increases the risk of DVT.
- A pre-operative assessment is completed.
- The options for definitive treatment of gallstones are discussed with the patient and their relatives.

This patient has two options. One is conservative management that is already in place. Alternatively, she can be offered an urgent laparoscopic cholecystectomy. This patient is obese; the response to uncontrolled infection in an obese patient is worse than a patient of average weight.

In the past, such patients were managed conservatively and offered elective cholecystectomy 6-8 weeks later. It was expected that during this period the inflammatory adhesions would resolve and so make the operation technically easier and safer.

With the advent of laparoscopic cholecystectomy, the management approach has shifted towards early surgery. The previous experience has been that some patients who were awaiting elective cholecystectomy would return with another episode of cholecystitis or complications such as cholangitis, pancreatitis or jaundice related to gallstones prior to surgery (Table 1). This was the main drawback of the conservative approach. Re-admission rates as high as 18-20% have been reported. The cost in ill health as well as financial considerations of re-admission have become important issues.

Many studies have confirmed the safety profile of laparoscopic cholecystectomy in the setting of acute cholecystitis. The present consensus is to regard emergency cholecystectomy as a safe option, if performed within 48-72 hours of the onset of acute cholecystitis, by an experienced surgeon. The evidence has emerged that the outcome of this approach is comparable, or even better, when compared with the traditional conservative approach.

The threshold for conversion from a laparoscopic to open procedure should be kept low when embarking on this approach. The experience of the surgeon and his mindset with the 'safety first' approach cannot be over-emphasised. The patient and their family should be given a clear and concise explanation as to the rationale of this approach, the necessity of having a low threshold for conversion, and all the recognised complications inherent to laparoscopic cholecystectomy in general and emergency laparoscopic cholecystectomy, particularly in an obese patient. The final decision should be made by the patient with a clear understanding of the risks and benefits of the approach.

Clinical points

- Bile duct injury is the most dreaded complication of laparoscopic cholecystectomy.
- The rate of bile duct injury following laparoscopic cholecystectomy is approximately twice that of open procedures.
- Bleeding, bile collection, infection, diathermy or instrumental injury to other organs and port-site herniae are the other possible procedure-specific complications.

Progress of the patient

- The patient decides to have an emergency laparoscopic cholecystectomy.
- Arrangements are made to perform an operative cholangiogram if deemed necessary but this is not performed.
- The postoperative period is uneventful.

Currently, opinion is divided as to whether routine cholangiograms should be performed in all patients undergoing a laparoscopic cholecystectomy. Proponents of routine cholangiography argue that its use helps to prevent bile duct injury, allows detection of bile duct calculi and is necessary for training purposes. Some advocate a selective policy of cholangiography, imaging only those considered to be at risk for choledocholithiasis. They argue that the studies in the literature using selective cholangiography have not shown a significant increase in the incidence of retained bile duct stones or biliary injury. The cholangiogram may add to the overall morbidity of the operation and may be difficult in an acute setting. This patient did not have clinical, biochemical or imaging evidence of bile duct stones and the anatomy was not difficult during the procedure; hence, a selective policy was adopted.

Suggested reading

1. UK guidelines for the management of acute pancreatitis. UK Working Party on Acute Pancreatitis. *Gut* 2005; 54: 1-9.
2. Yusoff. IF, Barkun JS, Barkun AN. Diagnosis and management of cholecystitis and cholangitis. *Gastroenterology Clinics of North America* 2003; 32: 1145-68.
3. Gurusamy KS, Samraj K. Early versus delayed laparoscopic cholecystectomy for acute cholecystitis. *Cochrane Database of Systematic Reviews* 2006; 4: CD005440.

Self-assessment

Q1
EMQ

a. Urgent laparoscopic cholecystectomy.
b. Urgent open cholecystectomy.
c. Conservative management.
d. Elective laparoscopic cholecystectomy.
e. Elective open cholecystectomy.
f. Low threshold for conversion.
g. High threshold for conversion.
h. A concise discussion of all recognised complications of surgery.

Select items relevant to the best management practice for the definitive management of gallbladder stones in the patient whose clinical presentation is described below.

A 60-year-old diabetic women presents with right hypochondrial pain of 2 days' duration. She is pyrexial. Abdominal examination reveals right hypochondrial tenderness and guarding. Her WCC is 14,000/mm^3. Serum amylase and liver enzyme levels are normal. An ultrasound scan reveals multiple gallstones, gallbladder wall oedema and a normal diameter bile duct.

Q2
EMQ

a. Mucocele of the gallbladder.
b. Gallstone pancreatitis.
c. Chronic cholecystitis.
d. Acute cholecystitis.
e. Empyema of the gallbladder.
f. Acute pyogenic cholangitis.
g. Biliary colic.
h. Obstructive jaundice.

Select the most likely clinical diagnosis from the conditions mentioned above for the case scenarios described below.

1. A 60-year-old multipara presents with recurrent dyspepsia and chronic right hypochondrial pain. Her BMI is 54.
2. A 35-year-old school teacher presents with severe excruciating right hypochondrial pain radiating round to her back. She responds to pethidine. The pain resolves completely after 6 hours. Her mother has had surgery for gallstone disease.
3. A 76-year-old man presents with fever with chills and rigors of 2 days' duration. He is known to have gallstones. He has dark urine and is icteric.
4. A 45-year-old male awaiting cholecystectomy for gallstones, is admitted with sudden onset of severe abdominal pain. He looks unwell and dehydrated. He has generalised abdominal tenderness and guarding.

Q3
SBA

A 60-year-old diabetic women presents with right hypochondrial pain of 2 days' duration. She is pyrexial and has right hypochondrial tenderness and guarding. Her WCC is 14,000/mm^3 and serum amylase and liver enzymes are normal. An ultrasound scan reveals multiple gallstones, gallbladder wall oedema and a normal diameter bile duct.

What is the most appropriate next step in the management of this patient?

a. Emergency laparoscopic cholecystectomy.
b. Emergency open cholecystectomy.
c. Intravenous broad-spectrum antibiotics and nil by mouth.
d. Transfer to ICU.
e. Urgent CT scan.
f. Urgent magnetic resonance cholangio-pancreatogram (MRCP).

Q4
True/False

a. Asymptomatic gallbladder stones are more common than symptomatic gallstones.
b. Mirizzi syndrome is caused by stones in the bile duct.
c. Gallstones are frequently found in stools in patients with gallstone pancreatitis.
d. Gallstone pancreatitis is more commonly seen in patients with small gallstones.
e. Open exploration of the bile duct is the treatment of choice for acute suppurative cholangitis.

Answers overleaf

Self-assessment answers

Q1 (a), (f), (h).

Explanatory notes

A diabetic with acute cholecystitis presenting within 48 hours of onset. Diabetics are more prone to develop severe biliary sepsis. Removal of the inflamed gallbladder by an experienced surgeon using the laparoscopic technique with a low threshold for conversion is the best evidence-based management practice.

Q2 1. (c) , 2. (g), 3. (f), 4. (b).

Q3 (c).

Q4 a. (T), b. (F), c. (T), d. (T), e. (F).

Explanatory notes

b. Mirizzi syndrome is due to a stone embedded in Hartmann's pouch which is adherent to the common hepatic duct. The resultant inflammation may produce a clinical picture compatible with bile duct obstruction, although the stone is not in the bile duct. Frequently, the inflammation causes obliteration of the anatomy of Calot's triangle and this makes the laparoscopic dissection of Calot's triangle hazardous. Many surgeons consider Mirizzi syndrome as a contraindication to proceed with the laparoscopic approach.

c, d. There is evidence that gallstone pancreatitis is frequently associated with multiple, small faceted stones, a wide patent cystic duct, presence of a common channel and stones which are a little too big to pass through the ampullary opening with ease, but not too big to obliterate the entire length of the common channel. The present evidence indicates that gallstone pancreatitis is initiated by the transient impaction of such a stone at the ampullary opening. This may allow the reflux of bile from the bile duct to the pancreatic duct behind the obstructing stone because there is a space in the common channel behind the stone for reflux to occur. Alternatively, the temporary obstruction to the ampullary opening may cause injury to the ampulla leading to sphincter dysfunction. The incompetent ampullary opening may allow activated pancreatic enzymes to reflux back to the pancreas to initiate pancreatitis. Pioneering work by Acosta and Ledesma by isolating stones in faeces in the majority of patients with gallstone pancreatitis during the first few days of an episode has given credit to the so called 'transient impaction and migration theory' of gallstone pancreatitis.

e. Urgent endoscopic drainage (endoscopic retrograde cholangiopancreatography [ERCP] and stenting) is the treatment of choice for acute suppurative cholangitis. Acute pyogenic cholangitis is characterised by Charcot's triad: fever, pain and jaundice. When gram negative organisms multiply in the obstructed bile duct the infection will ascend to the largest vascular organ in the human body, the liver. Gram negative septicaemia and toxaemia will soon follow. Acute toxic cholangitis is the most dangerous form, where there is hypotension and confusion. The mortality of untreated toxic cholangitis is almost 100%. ERCP and drainage of the duct can be life-saving.

Chapter 5

Obstructive jaundice

Learning objectives

- To learn the clinical approach to work out the level and cause of jaundice in a patient with suspected extrahepatic biliary obstruction.
- To learn the initial work-up to establish a diagnosis.
- To be familiar with the different investigative modalities and their principles.
- To work out the best management plan based on the pathological and radiological evidence.
- To be familiar with the anatomical basis of surgery for pancreatic cancer.
- To learn the value and limitations of pre-operative biliary drainage.

Case scenario

A 72-year-old male presents with a 1-month history of generalised weakness and loss of appetite. About 3 weeks previously he noticed that his urine has become dark which he attributed to drinking less water. His wife noticed a change in the colour of his skin and the primary care physician found that he was jaundiced. One week before presenting to the hospital, he developed pruritus which had become troublesome especially at night. On direct questioning he admits that his stools have become pale. He develops abdominal discomfort after meals but denies having abdominal pain. He had been a heavy smoker but gave up 10 years ago. He has consumed about two bottles of wine a week for the last 5 years. He has no other significant comorbidities.

On examination he appears unwell, slightly dehydrated, thin and obviously icteric. There is no lymphadenopathy. No stigmata of chronic liver disease are evident. Abdominal examination reveals a firm liver edge 3cm below the right costal margin with the upper border of the liver at the fifth rib level on percussion. A tensely cystic mass which moves on respiration is palpable in the right hypochondrium. There is no clinical evidence of free fluid in the abdomen and the digital rectal examination is normal.

The most likely clinical diagnosis: obstructive jaundice.

Jaundice becomes clinically apparent when the bilirubin level reaches 40mmol/l. Scleral elastin has a high affinity for bilirubin, and with a white background, it is a sensitive indicator of jaundice. This is the reason why jaundice is easily detectable in the eyes. Dark urine confirms conjugated hyperbilirubinaemia which is filtered via the kidneys. Unconjugated bilirubin is tightly bound to albumin which prevents glomerular filtration. Deposition of bile salts irritates the skin and causes pruritus. Stools are pale because the bile is not reaching the duodenum.

The most likely cause of jaundice in this patient is a malignant obstruction of the extrahepatic biliary tree. Painless progressive obstructive jaundice in the elderly is highly suggestive of a malignant obstruction.

The most likely level of the obstruction is below the insertion of the cystic duct. When the common bile duct is obstructed and the cystic duct is patent and accessible, the bile, instead of passing into the duodenum will continue to fill and distend the gallbladder. That is why this patient has a palpable gallbladder. If the bile duct is obstructed in the region of the common hepatic duct then the bile will not reach the gallbladder or the duodenum. Such patients will have jaundice but will not have a palpable gallbladder.

Clinical points

- Jaundice, pale stools, dark urine and pruritus are the classical clinical features of an obstruction to the extrahepatic biliary tree.
- Progressive painless obstructive jaundice in the elderly is highly suspicious of a malignant obstruction.

Could the obstruction be due to a stone in the bile duct and not due to a cancer?

It is very unlikely due to two reasons:

- An obstructing bile duct stone classically presents with a history of severe epigastric pain. This patient has painless obstructive jaundice.
- Most bile duct stones are formed in the gallbladder and will reach the bile duct after escaping through the cystic duct. This will take time and gallstones are often present in the gallbladder for months or years. During this period, the gallbladder wall reacts to the presence of stones. The wall of the gallbladder becomes thickened and contracted due to a chronic inflammatory reaction. This patient has a tensely cystic globular structure in the right hypochondrium, which clinically is a distended gallbladder. This physical sign is against stone disease as the cause of biliary obstruction. This is because a contracted thick-walled gallbladder will not distend sufficiently for it to become clinically palpable. This clinical picture is consistent with 'Courvoisier's law'.

Clinical points

- Courvoisier's law: in a patient who is jaundiced and has a palpable gallbladder, the cause of the obstruction is unlikely to be due to a stone in the bile duct.

In 1890, Courvoisier presented his observation that a palpable gallbladder in a patient with obstructive jaundice is often caused by a non-calculus abnormality of the hepatobiliary system (e.g. pancreatic cancer or stricture of the common bile duct). When this observation came to be referred to as a 'law' is not clear. This observation has also been referred to as Courvoisier's sign or Courvoisier's gallbladder but Courvoisier never coined these words.

Is it possible that this patient may have a mucocele of the gallbladder due to a stone obstructing the cystic duct and another stone in the bile duct causing obstructive jaundice at the same time?

It is possible, but this is a very rare occurrence. A mucocele results when a stone obstructs a relatively empty gallbladder which becomes filled with mucus secreted by the abnormally active mucous glands in response to wall contractions. A mucocele of the gallbladder is an uncommon finding, but another stone resulting in bile duct obstruction causing jaundice at the same time would be a very rare coincidence. In medicine it is rare to find two uncommon occurrences presenting at the same time.

Could the level of obstruction be higher such as at the porta hepatis?

It is very unlikely because his gallbladder is palpable. This physical sign indicates that bile reaches the gallbladder but cannot drain to the duodenum when required. Therefore, the block must be below the site of entry of the cystic duct to the bile duct.

There are two conditions that should be considered when a jaundiced patient is found to have a dilated intrahepatic biliary tree on ultrasound with no clinical or ultrasound evidence of dilatation of the extrahepatic biliary tree. The two conditions are cholangio-carcinoma of the common hepatic duct (also referred to as Klatskin's tumour) and malignant nodes at the porta hepatis obstructing the common hepatic duct. A cancer of the gallbladder can also invade this level of the extrahepatic biliary tree and produce a similar picture but generally a gallbladder growth tends to be picked up by an ultrasound scan.

Does absence of pain exclude the possibility of a bile duct stone causing obstructive jaundice?

It is well known that obstruction to the bile duct or cystic duct will cause severe upper abdominal pain. However, it is also recognised that some elderly patients with large bile duct stones may present with obstructive jaundice without pain, but they will not have a palpable gallbladder. This patient has a palpable gallbladder with painless obstructive jaundice.

What is the differential diagnosis?

Possible causes of malignant obstruction to the bile duct below the insertion of the cystic duct are:

- Carcinoma of the head of the pancreas.
- Carcinoma of the ampulla of Vater.
- Cholangiocarcinoma of the distal common bile duct.

What other leading questions may help to make the diagnosis?

Presence of melaena

Ampullary cancers (Figure 1) may bleed and cause intermittent melaena. This is because when the cancer expands it occludes the lumen of the ampulla which causes an increase in the bile duct pressure, due to the stagnation of bile. The stagnation of bile will exert pressure on the tumour tissue and bile flow will break through the tumour. Tumours have fragile blood vessels and they bleed easily. This will lessen the extent of jaundice and will also produce melaena.

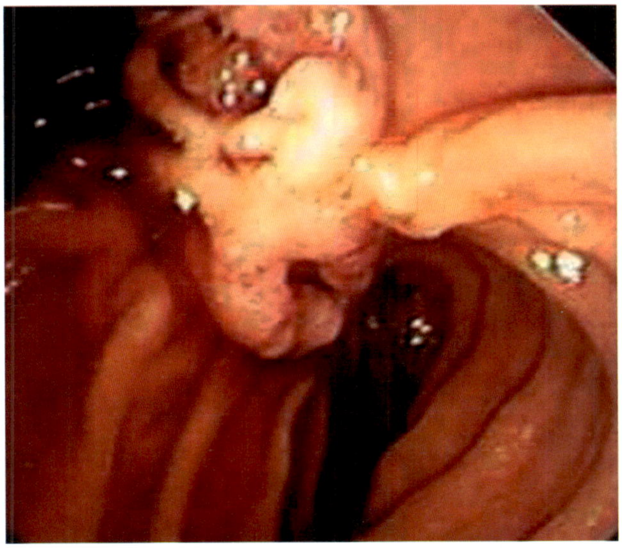

Figure 1. Endoscopic view of a peri-ampullary cancer. *Reproduced with permission from Hans Bjorknas, Gastrolab, Finland. www.gastrolab.net.*

Back pain and weight loss

Significant involuntary weight loss associated with back pain preceding the appearance of jaundice supports a diagnosis of cancer of the head of the pancreas.

Progress of the patient

- Haematological and biochemical assessments are performed:
  - haemoglobin (Hb) 11.1g/dL;
  - bilirubin 40μmol/L (0.3-18μmol/L);
  - alanine transaminase (ALT) 98U/L (5-45 U/L (international units per litre);
  - aspartate transaminase (AST) 80U/L (5-45U/L);
  - alkaline phosphatase (ALP) 430U/L (30-120U/L);
  - gamma glutamyl transpeptidase (GGT) 400U/L (5-35U/L);
  - urea 1.3mmol/L (2.5-6.4mmol/L);
  - creatinine 108mmol/L (94-110mmol/L);
  - prothrombin time 8 sec (10-15 seconds);
  - International Normalisation Ratio (INR) 1.2 (1-1.3);
  - tumour markers - CA 19-9 40U/ml (0-37U/ml);
- An ultrasound scan shows a markedly distended thin-walled gallbladder. There is dilatation of the intrahepatic biliary tree and the bile duct is dilated to 1.3cm (normal up to 7mm). This is noted up to the distal end. A mass lesion is identified in the pancreatic head.
- A CT scan is performed, which confirms a 2.5cm x 2.5cm mass lesion in the region of the pancreatic head, not involving the superior mesenteric vein or portal vein. Three enlarged lymph nodes are seen in the retroperitoneum adjacent to the pancreas.

The radiological finding of a dilated intrahepatic biliary tree is significant. Unlike the extrahepatic bile duct, the intrahepatic biliary tree may not become dilated with ease. This is because of its intraparenchymal position. For dilatation of the intrahepatic biliary tree to occur against resistance there must be significant occlusion of the bile duct. This means that either there is a malignant infiltration or a benign fibrotic lesion causing stenosis. Most such benign strictures are due to iatrogenic bile duct injuries or strictures following repair of such injuries.

It is not uncommon to observe deep jaundice in patients with a dilated extrahepatic biliary tree. If such a patient is found to have a dilated intrahepatic biliary tree with no history of previous surgery and no ultrasound evidence of stones in the gallbladder or bile duct, it is very likely that the patient may have a malignant obstruction in the extrahepatic biliary tree or in the pancreatic head.

One of the challenges in the diagnosis of such a clinical presentation is the difficulty in obtaining a tissue diagnosis even after accurately defining the level of occlusion. The so called Klatskin's tumour, cholangiocarcinoma of the common hepatic duct, is a classic example. During endoscopic retrograde cholangiopancreatography (ERCP), the endoscopist will perform brush cytology by introducing an endoscopic brush into the common hepatic duct to the site of the tumour. The diagnostic yield of ERCP and brush cytology can be disappointingly low even in expert hands.

This patient has a pancreatic head mass.

What is the next step?

- To obtain a histological diagnosis of the pancreatic head mass.
- An endoscopic ultrasound (EUS) is performed, which confirms the hypoechoic mass with a relatively unclear margin and irregular internal echos suggestive of cancer. There is no evidence of vascular invasion. Endoscopic ultrasound-guided biopsy confirms a pancreatic adenocarcinoma.

What is endoscopic ultrasound?

The principle is the same as ultrasound but the ultrasound probe is attached to the end of a side-viewing duodenoscope (ERCP scope). The scope is then positioned in the duodenum close to the lesion using the same technique as in ERCP. Because the probe is placed very close to the lesion, clear views and biopsy specimens can be obtained.

Compared with conventional ultrasonography, ERCP and computed tomography (CT), endoscopic ultrasonography (EUS) has the highest detection rates for tumours of the pancreas, especially in detecting small tumours.

EUS is also valuable for the detection of vascular invasion.

Progress of the patient

- The patient is discussed at the MDT meeting. CT data are suggestive of an operable tumour. The patient has no significant comorbid factors to preclude radical excisional surgery.
- The decision is made to perform a Whipple operation. Intra-operative laparoscopy is planned in order to assess for any small peritoneal deposits before commencement of the curative resection.

Pancreatic cancer is one of the most aggressive cancers with an extremely poor prognosis. Radical resection offers the only chance of cure. However, due to the aggressiveness of the cancer, most patients are found to have distant metastases or retroperitoneal infiltration at the time of diagnosis. About 70% occur in the head of the pancreas. Head tumours present with the effects of bile duct obstruction. Those in the body and tail present late and are very rarely suitable for curative surgery.

Overall survival rates after curative intent surgery remains dismally low at around 5%, although some centres have reported 5-year survival rates of 20% for early cancers.

Therefore, identification of patients who could be offered radical curative intent surgery is very important and the decision should be made by a multidisciplinary team.

Resectability criteria for pancreatic head cancers include the:

- Absence of vascular involvement. Identification of a clear fat plane around the coeliac and superior mesenteric arteries, and a patent superior mesenteric vein and portal vein.
- Absence of small peritoneal or hepatic deposits at diagnostic laparoscopy. Approximately 20-40% of patients may be found to be unsuitable for curative intent resection due to the presence of small peritoneal or hepatic metastases not visualised by CT but recognised at laparoscopy prior to major surgery.
- Absence of distant metastases. Important prognostic features include tumour size (<2cm), lymph node involvement and histological grading.

What is a Whipple operation?

This is a major complex operation which involves the removal of the head, the neck and part of the body of the pancreas, distal one third of the stomach, the duodenum, part of the common bile duct and the gallbladder. Some surgeons preserve the pylorus and therefore the stomach is not removed (pylorus-preserving pancreatoduodenectomy [PPPD]). The jejunum is used for reconstruction

The procedure carries a significant morbidity and mortality. Mortality of this procedure has declined from 20% to 1-5% in centres regularly performing pancreatic surgery. However, the morbidity rate remains unchanged. The main cause of morbidity and mortality of this operation is related to pancreatic fistulae due to leaks from the pancreatojejunal anastomosis.

Other postoperative complications include delayed gastric emptying, splenic vein thrombosis, infection and bleeding.

Why is endoscopic retrograde cholangiopancreatography (ERCP) not considered in this patient?

To perform an ERCP a side-viewing duodenoscope is used to visualise the ampulla which is cannulated and contrast is injected to outline the pancreatobiliary tree. The main drawback of ERCP is that about 2-5% of patients will develop post-ERCP pancreatitis. Endoscopic ultrasound (EUS) is also performed with the same endoscope with the ultrasound probe attached to its end. Before the ultrasound probe is activated, endoscopic views of the stomach, duodenum and ampulla can be obtained. No abnormality was demonstrated on the endoscopic views of this patient. Therefore, ERCP was not considered, as EUS and the CT scan provided the same information without the risk of post-ERCP pancreatitis.

What is pre-operative biliary drainage and why is it not considered in this patient?

Before definitive surgery, the bile can be drained by placing a drain percutaneously or by placing a stent in the bile duct through the ampulla across the site of the obstruction using the ERCP scope. The role of pre-operative biliary drainage is controversial due to the fact that although it might relieve the jaundice and attendant biochemical abnormalities, some recent studies have identified increased septic complications especially during the immediate postoperative period.

This patient is not septic and surgery is planned early. Therefore, pre-operative biliary drainage is not considered.

If it is decided to drain the biliary tree pre-operatively, there are two methods available:

- Percutaneous transhepatic biliary drainage (PTBD).
- Endoscopic biliary stenting.

PTBD

An external drain is inserted to the dilated intrahepatic biliary tree under ultrasound guidance and the bile is drained to a bag. This technique will relieve the biliary obstruction but does not restore bile flow to the intestine.

Endoscopic biliary stenting

Using a side-viewing duodenoscope, the ampulla is cannulated and a plastic stent (7F or 10F) is placed in the bile duct. This technique will relieve the biliary obstruction and restore bile flow to the intestine. It is also a very useful technique for palliation.

Progress of the patient

- The patient is discharged home on the tenth postoperative day following an uncomplicated Whipple operation.
- Eighteen months after the Whipple operation the patient is admitted as an emergency. He looks unwell and anaemic with marked abdominal distension. He has ascites. A CT scan reveals massive ascites and widespread intraperitoneal cancer. A palliative care team is summoned and he is treated with narcotic analgesics. He passes away peacefully, 20 months following surgery.

Of all cancers of the gastrointestinal system, pancreatic cancer has the worst prognosis. Surgery is considered as the mainstay of treatment but the resectability rate is low due to advanced stage at the time of presentation. The results of neoadjuvant and adjuvant treatments have historically been disappointing. However, a landmark trial in 2007 using gemcitabine as adjuvant chemotherapy following resection of pancreatic cancer showed a survival benefit regardless of resection margin or nodal status and established postoperative gemcitabine as the standard of care. Gemcitabine is also considered by many centres as the current standard therapy for metastatic pancreatic adenocarcinoma.

Suggested reading

1. Guidelines for the management of patients with pancreatic cancer. Periampullary and ampullary carcinomas. *Gut* 2005; 54 suppl 5: v1-16.
2. Oettle H, *et al.* Adjuvant chemotherapy with gemcitabine vs observation in patients undergoing curative-intent resection of pancreatic cancer: a randomized controlled trial. *JAMA* 2007; 297: 267-77.
3. Burris HA 3rd, Moore MJ, Andersen J, Green MR, Rothenberg ML, Modiano MR, Cripps MC, Portenoy RK, Storniolo AM, Tarassoff P, Nelson R, Dorr FA, Stephens CD, Von Hoff DD. Improvements in survival and clinical benefit with gemcitabine as first-line therapy for patients with advanced pancreas cancer: a randomized trial. *J Clin Oncol* 1997; 15(6): 2403-13.

Self-assessment

Q1
EMQ

a. Acute cholecystitis.
b. Acute pancreatitis.
c. Acute cholangitis.
d. Biliary colic.
e. Mucocele of the gallbladder.
f. Cancer of the ampulla of Vater.
g. Chronic cholecystitis.
h. Choledochoduodenal fistula.

Select the most likely clinical diagnosis from the conditions mentioned above for the case scenarios described below.

1. A 72-year-old male presents with jaundice, pale stools, dark urine and pruritus. He has a palpable gallbladder.
2. One week after an episode of right hypochondrial pain which lasted for 24 hours, a 55-year-old female presents with a palpable lump in the right hypochondrium. She looks well and is not icteric.
3. A 55-year-old female awaiting cholecystectomy for symptomatic gallstone disease presents with severe central abdominal pain of 24 hours' duration. She looks ill, dehydrated and has generalised abdominal tenderness and guarding.
4. A 70-year-old male awaiting cholecystectomy for symptomatic gallstone disease presents with epigastric pain and fever with chills and rigors. He is slightly icteric.
5. An obese 40-year-old mother of five presents with a 4-month history of intermittent dyspepsia and upper abdominal pain.

Q2
SBA

A 55-year-old man presents with painless obstructive jaundice of 1 month's duration. He has a palpable cystic mass in the right hypochondrium which on ultrasound is confirmed to be a distended gallbladder. Ultrasound has also detected a mass in the pancreatic head.

What is the most appropriate next step in the management of this patient?

a. Abdominal CT scan and biopsy.
b. Endoscopic ultrasound and a biopsy.
c. ERCP.
d. MRCP.
e. CA19.9.

Q3
SBA

A 77-year-old man is diagnosed as having metastatic pancreatic cancer. He is deeply icteric and has severe itching.

What is the most appropriate therapy for this patient?

a. Radiation treatment to the pancreatic cancer.
b. Placement of a metal stent in the bile duct.
c. Cholestyramine.
d. Surgical bypass procedure.
e. Tender loving care.

Q4
True/False

An ultrasound scan performed on a deeply icteric elderly male reveals a dilated intrahepatic biliary tree. The gallbladder and bile duct are not visualised.

The likely causes of the obstruction will include:

a. Cholangiocarcinoma of the common hepatic duct.
b. Cholangiocarcinoma of the distal common bile duct.
c. Enlarged lymph nodes at the porta hepatis causing compression.
d. Carcinoma of the head of the pancreas.
e. Carcinoma of the ampulla of Vater.

Q5
True/False

The possible sites of obstruction in a patient with painless obstructive jaundice, a palpable gallbladder and dilatation of the intrahepatic biliary tree on ultrasound would be the:

a. Common bile duct.
b. Common hepatic duct.
c. Cystic duct.
d. Porta hepatis.
e. Ampulla of Vater.

Q6
True/False

a. The majority of pancreatic cancers are unresectable at presentation.
b. Conjugated hyperbilirubinaemia is associated with pancreatic head cancers.
c. Suppurative cholangitis is associated with bile duct stones.
d. Retained bile duct stones found after open cholecystectomy are best managed with endoscopic sphincterotomy and stone extraction.
e. The Whipple operation is associated with long-term survival rates for pancreatic head cancer when performed with a curative intent.

Answers overleaf

Self-assessment answers

Q1 1. (f), 2. (e), 3. (b), 4. (c), 5. (g).

Q2 (b).

Explanatory notes

Endoscopic ultrasound provides the best opportunity to obtain accurate tumour characteristics and a representative sample for histology.

Q3 (b).

Explanatory notes

Palliative biliary drainage with a self-expandable metal stent is a minimally invasive procedure that is performed under sedation. It has been shown to be the best outcome-based therapy for the relief of jaundice and pruritus in such patients.

Q4 a. (T), b. (F), c. (T), d. (F), e. (F).

Q5 a. (T), b. (F), c. (F), d. (F), e. (T).

Q6 a. (T), b. (T), c. (T), d. (T) e. (F).

Chapter 6

Acute pancreatitis

Learning objectives

- To learn the initial management of acute pancreatitis.
- To learn the course and pathophysiology of acute pancreatitis.
- To understand the importance of differentiating between acute mild and acute severe pancreatitis.
- To understand the value and limitations of the prognostic indices of acute pancreatitis.
- To learn the role of ERCP and endoscopic sphincterotomy in the management of acute biliary pancreatitis.

Case scenario

A 61-year-old obese female presents with severe abdominal pain of 24-hour duration. The pain began suddenly after lunch on the previous day. The pain is constant, located in the upper part of the abdomen and radiates through to the back. At night she vomited a large amount but this did not relieve her pain.

Her past medical history is unremarkable. She consumes alcohol occasionally and she is a non-smoker. She has no history of diabetes.

On examination, the patient appears to be in pain. Her temperature is 38°C, heart rate is 110/minute, blood pressure (BP) is 110/70mm Hg and respiratory rate (RR) is 28/minute.

The abdomen is distended and is tender to palpation in the epigastrium. Bowel sounds are present but reduced.

The most likely clinical diagnosis: acute pancreatitis.

The suddenness of the onset, the severity and the location of the pain raise the possibility of an obstructive lesion in a tubular structure in the region. The tubular structures to be considered are the cystic duct, bile duct and pancreatic duct. The other possibility is a leak from an organ in that vicinity into the peritoneal cavity.

Pyrexia, tachycardia, tachypnoea and epigastric tenderness suggest the onset of an acute inflammatory condition in the upper abdomen.

The most likely organ systems are:

- Biliary and pancreatic system.
- Upper gastrointestinal (GI) tract (stomach and duodenum).

The most likely clinical diagnosis in this patient is acute pancreatitis.

This patient has a history of severe upper abdominal pain radiating through to the back and tenderness over the anatomical region of the pancreas. In the absence of a history of alcohol consumption, the most likely aetiology of acute pancreatitis is gallstones.

The raised amylase and lipase levels and the evidence of a pancreatic swelling on the abdominal ultrasound/CT scan will confirm the diagnosis.

Differential diagnoses to be considered are as follows.

Could this clinical picture be due to biliary colic leading to acute cholecystitis?

Biliary colic is characterised by the sudden onset of severe right hypochondrial pain radiating round to the back. This is caused by a gallstone obstructing the cystic duct and the gallbladder contracting against the obstruction to empty it. Although the classical site of biliary colic pain is the right hypochondrium, it is not unusual for patients with biliary colic to present with epigastric pain.

If the obstruction is not relieved, the stagnated bile in the gallbladder will become infected. This condition is called acute cholecystitis. Persistence of pain, fever, tachycardia and epigastric tenderness are further supportive evidence of an infection in the gallbladder. Although the right hypochondrium is the classic site of tenderness in acute cholecystitis, the site of tenderness will depend on the location of the inflamed gallbladder.

Gallbladder stones, wall oedema and/or fluid around the gallbladder on imaging will be evidence of acute suppurative cholecystitis.

Is the clinical picture compatible with acute cholangitis?

The obstruction of the bile duct can be caused by a gallstone which has escaped from the gallbladder to the bile duct. This causes stasis of bile. Whenever there is stasis in the biliary tree, infection will follow which results in cholangitis.

Fever, tachycardia, tachypnoea, mild jaundice and epigastric tenderness supports a diagnosis of acute cholangitis. The imaging evidence of dilatation of the bile duct and the presence of bile duct stones provide other supportive evidence.

Biliary pancreatitis can be complicated by acute pyogenic cholangitis when there is significant obstruction to the bilary tree. High fever with chills and sometimes with rigors is characteristic of acute pyogenic cholangitis. This is not seen in this patient.

Could this be due to a perforated peptic ulcer?

The commonest condition which causes a leak of contents into the peritoneal cavity in the upper abdomen is the perforation of a chronic peptic ulcer. However, this patient has no history suggestive of peptic ulcer disease. It would be unusual for her to have a silent peptic ulcer perforation. Silent peptic ulcers (peptic ulcers without symptoms) are usually seen in elderly patients who are on long-term non-steroidal anti-inflammatory drug (NSAID) therapy or on steroids but this patient has no such history.

Progress of the patient

- Results of investigations:
  - WCC 17,000/mm^3;
  - Hb 15g/dL;
  - haematocrit 0.47;
  - fasting blood glucose 12mmol/L (4-7mmol/L);
  - bilirubin 20μmol/L (0.3-18μmol/L);
  - AST 350U/L (5-45U/L);
  - ALT 430U/L (5-45U/L);
  - Lactate dehydrogenase (LDH) 300U/L;
  - S amylase 6000U/L (23-85U/L);
  - S calcium 1.9mmol/L (2.2-2.6mmol/L);
  - pH 7.3 (7.35-7.45);
  - PCO_2 33mm Hg (35-45mm Hg);
  - PaO_2 68mmHg (80-100mm Hg);
  - HCO_3 21mmol/L;
  - C-reactive protein (CRP) 80mg/L;
  - INR 1.2;
  - S creatinine 108mmol/l (94-110mmol/L);
- The chest X-ray shows a small pleural effusion.

Clinical points

- Serum amylase more than three times the upper limit of normal is diagnostic of acute pancreatitis.
- Fever, tachypnoea, tachycardia, leucocytosis, an increased haematocrit (haemoconcentration), hypocalcaemia, raised blood glucose in a patient who is not a known diabetic, raised CRP, raised LDH and AST, hypoxaemia and pleural effusion suggest the onset of acute severe pancreatitis.
- Age and obesity are other potential risk factors in this patient.

What is the next step?

- The patient is transferred to a high dependency unit (HDU) for close monitoring.
- Oxygen is given by mask and monitored by a pulse oximeter.
- An IV infusion is set up with normal (N) saline 2-4-hourly.
- The patient is catheterised and the rate of intravenous infusion is maintained to achieve an hourly urine output of 30ml or above
- If the urine output falls below 30ml per hour, despite increasing intravenous fluids, a central venous pressure (CVP) line should be inserted for close monitoring of the haemodynamic status.
- A contrast-enhanced CT scan is performed, the findings of which are:
  - multiple small gallstones in the gallbladder;
  - an oedematous pancreas with a small peri-pancreatic fluid collection;
  - no evidence of pancreatic necrosis;
  - a dilated bile duct 9.6mm (normal 6-7mm);
  - no stones in the bile duct noted.
- The diagnosis is acute severe pancreatitis due to gallstones.

Clinical points

- There is evidence that the outcome of patients with acute severe pancreatitis is improved by intensive monitoring and aggressive therapy. According to British Society of Gastroenterology (BSG) guidelines, all patients with suspected severe pancreatitis should be managed in a HDU or intensive care unit (ICU) setting.

What is the role of an abdominal ultrasound scan? Why is a CT scan and not an ultrasound scan requested as the first imaging investigation for this patient?

UK guidelines for the management of acute pancreatitis suggest that all patients with acute pancreatitis must have an ultrsound scan within 24 hours of admission to exclude gallstones. An ultrasound scan is very sensitive in identifying gallbladder stones. However, it is not a very sensitive investigation to identify early changes in the pancreas. This patient has clinical and biochemical evidence suggestive of acute severe pancreatitis. Therefore, an early contrast CT will be useful to identify and document the changes of the pancreas. It will also be useful as a baseline, if the condition of the patient deteriorates to pancreatic necrosis. For a patient with no evidence of acute severe pancreatitis, an abdominal ultrasound scan will be the first imaging investigation.

Clinical points

- Pyrexia, raised bilirubin, fever, a raised WCC and AST, and a dilated bile duct suggest the possibility of biliary sepsis with small stones or gravel in the bile duct.
- In the acute setting a CT/ultrasound scan can miss small bile duct stones.

What is acute severe pancreatitis?

In about 80% of patients with acute pancreatitis, inflammation of the pancreas will resolve completely with no long-term sequelae. This is known as acute mild pancreatitis. But 20% will develop multiple organ failure due to a systemic inflammatory response.

Multiple organ failure may also result from pancreatic necrosis with infection, which will lead to systemic and local complications. This is known as acute severe pancreatitis.

The difficulty is in recognising patients who are likely to develop acute severe pancreatitis at an early stage of the disease.

Why do these two types of acute pancreatitis have different outcomes?

The natural history of acute pancreatitis is unpredictable. Recollecting the pathophysiology of acute pancreatitis is important to understand why these two clinical groups have different outcomes. The pathogenesis of acute pancreatitis is divided into two phases.

The first phase, which commences from the time of onset of the pain, lasts for about a week or so. The severity of the first phase is related to multiple organ failure secondary to the extent of the host's systemic inflammatory response elicited by the tissue injury and not necessarily to the extent of the local pancreatic tissue damage. During this phase, there is oedema of the pancreas with a variable degree of pancreatic ischaemia. This is pathologically referred to as interstitial oedematous pancreatitis (IED).

Over the first week, the organ failure related to the systemic inflammatory response will either resolve or become more severe. Therefore, mortality during the first week is mostly related to the systemic inflammatory response leading to multiple organ failure and not due to local problems.

During the second phase, oedema of the pancreas will either resolve or progress to irreversible necrosis of the pancreas. This is pathologically referred to as necrotising pancreatitis. The necrosis is initially sterile but later becomes infected when the necrotic tissue is contaminated by translocated bacteria from the bowel.

Bacterial translocation means that the bacteria which are usually present inside the bowel migrate through the bowel wall due to changes in bowel permiability, contaminate the peritoneal cavity and infect the necrotic pancreas. The infection also can originate from pyogenic cholangitis due to biliary obstruction.

Necrotising pancreatitis may take a protracted course leading to many local complications. These include pancreatic fluid collections, peri-pancreatic abscesses, pancreatic ascites, pancreatic ductal disruptions, splenic or portal vein thrombosis and haemorrhage due to erosion of blood vessels.

A localised fluid collection after 4 weeks may develop into a cyst covered with a well developed wall around it and is referred to as a pancreatic pseudocyst.

Mortality during the second phase is usually related to whether or not necrosis becomes infected and the severity of the local and/or systemic infection. In general, necrotising pancreatitis is complicated by infection in approximately 50% of patients. Therefore, it is important to identify patients who are likely to develop acute severe pancreatitis at an early stage and to commence aggressive ICU-based resuscitation.

How to recognise patients who are likely to develop acute severe pancreatitis

Several prognostic systems have been developed to differentiate between acute mild pancreatitis and acute severe pancreatitis. These are:

- Ranson's criteria (Table 1).
- Glasgow Prognostic Score (Table 2).
- Acute Physiology And Chronic Health Evaluation (APACHE II) score.
- Balthazar score.

Ranson's criteria (Table 1) include five criteria on admission and six criteria after 48 hours. The Glasgow Prognostic Score (Table 2) is done only on admission. In both these systems, the presence of any three factors or more indicates acute severe pancreatitis.

Acute Physiology And Chronic Health Evaluation (APACHE II) score

APACHE II is designed to measure the severity of the disease in patients admitted to intensive care units. It provides a morbidity and mortality score. A point score is calculated from 12 routine physiological measurements (such as BP, heart rate, temperature, etc.) during the first 24 hours after admission, other information about health status of the patient and the patient's age.

Table 1. Ranson's criteria.

Present on admission

- Age >55.
- WCC >16,000/mm^3.
- Glucose >200mg/dL.
- LDH >350U/L.
- AST >250U/L.

Developing during the first 48 hours

- Haematocrit fall >10%.
- Blood urea nitrogen (BUN) >10%.
- S calcium <8mg/dL (2mmol/L).
- Arterial PaO_2 <60mm Hg.
- Base excess >4meq/L.
- Fluid sequestration >6L.

Score:
- <2 - predicted mortality 2%;
- 3-4 - predicted mortality 15%;
- 5-6 - predicted mortality 40%.

Table 2. Glasgow Prognostic Score.

- Age >55.
- WCC >15 x 10^9/L.
- Urea >16mmol/L.
- PaO_2 <60mm Hg.
- Albumin <32g/L.
- Calcium <2mmol/L.
- LDH >600U/L.
- AST/ALT >200U/L.

A score is calculated during the first 24 hours of admission. No new score is calculated after that. A chart for the calculation is available on-line. More than 8 points predicts 11-18% mortality.

Balthazar score

This score is based on the contrast-enhanced CT scan:

The score is from A to E:

- A to C - no mortality.
- E - 17% mortality.

C-reactive protein (CRP) is also recognised as a useful marker to predict acute severe pancreatitis. A CRP over 150mg/L indicates severe pancreatitis. This is easy to perform and is cheap. The main disadvantage is that it is an effective assessment tool only after 48 hours.

In reality, there is a wide variation in the use of different scoring systems. This highlights the lack of a universally accepted stratification system.

Progress of the patient

- Intravenous imipenum 1g b.d. is commenced.
- The contrast CT scan confirms acute biliary pancreatitis with no evidence of pancreatic necrosis.
- An ERCP and endoscopic sphincterotomy is performed. Multiple small stones are extracted with a biliary balloon and bile duct sweeping is done.
- A pancreatogram is not performed.
- Intensive monitoring in the ICU is continued with nasogastric aspiration and aggressive fluid resuscitation.
- The patient is feeling better after the ERCP and endoscopic biliary decompression.
- On the third day of admission, all haematological and biochemical investigations show improvement of her condition. Therefore, early enteral feeding is commenced via a nasogastric tube.

Use of antibiotics in the management of acute pancreatitis is controversial but many clinicians use it especially in patients with acute severe pancreatitis. There is evidence that antibiotics will improve the outcome in this group. Imipenum is effective as it penetrates pancreatic tissue well.

There is evidence that ERCP within the first 48 hours improves the outcome and mortality of patients with acute severe biliary pancreatitis. UK guidelines for the management of acute pancreatitis suggest that all patients with acute severe biliary pancreatitis must undergo ERCP and endoscopic sphincterotomy within 48 hours, especially if there is evidence of biliary sepsis.

In the past 'resting the pancreas' was the concept of treatment but there is evidence that early enteral feeding improves gut function, reduces bacterial translocation from the gut and reduces infective complications of pancreatitis.

Clinical points

- Imipenum is very effective as it penetrates pancreatic tissue.
- There is evidence that ERCP within the first 48 hours improves the outcome and mortality of patients with acute severe biliary pancreatitis.
- Early enteral feeding improves gut function, reduces bacterial translocation and reduces infective complications.

Progress of the patient

- Laparoscopic cholecystectomy is performed prior to discharge.
- The postoperative period is uneventful.

Recurrent attacks of acute pancreatitis occur in up to one out of three patients who do not undergo cholecystectomy.

This patient responded to urgent biliary decompression. However, if the patient's general condition had deteriorated, what would have been the next step?

The contrast CT scan should be repeated. If this demonstrates pancreatic necrosis (shown as an area of non-enhancement in Figure 1), the extent of the necrosis should be defined and needle aspiration should be performed under CT guidance. If the culture confirms infected pancreatic necrosis, under the appropriate antibiotic cover, the patient should be considered for pancreatic necrosectomy.

Pancreatic necrosectomy is a major complex procedure with a high morbidity and mortality. The decision to proceed to surgery should be supported by the MDT involving anaesthetists and ICU clinicians.

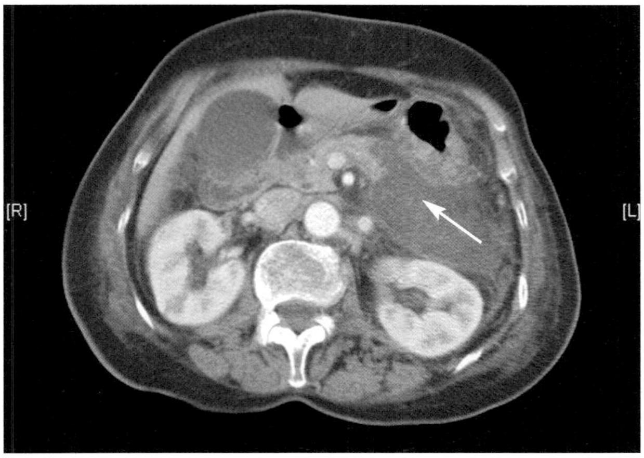

Figure 1. Contrast CT film with evidence of pancreatic necrosis (arrow). ***Reproduced with permission from Dr John Scally, Consultant Radiologist, Leighton Hospital, Crewe, Cheshire, UK.***

Suggested reading

1. UK guidelines for the management of acute pancreatitis. UK Working Party on Acute Pancreatitis. *Gut* 2005; 54: 1-9.
2. Williams ET, Green J, Beckingham I, Parks R, Martin D, Lombard M. Guidelines on the management of common bile duct stones. *Gut* 2008; 57(7): 1004-21.
3. Acute Physiology And Chronic Health Evaluation (APACHE II) score. Available at http://www.surgical-tutor.org.uk.

Self-assessment

Q1 EMQ

a. Pancreatic calcification.
b. Pancreatic necrosis.
c. Pancreatic divisum.
d. Occluding ampullary stone.

Match the type of pancreatitis most associated with the pancreatobiliary abnormality mentioned above.

1. Acute biliary pancreatitis.
2. Recurrent acute pancreatitis.
3. Chronic pancreatitis.
4. Acute severe pancreatitis.

Q2 SBA

A 58-year-old heavy alcoholic male presents with constant severe upper abdominal pain of 3 days' duration. The abdomen is distended with marked tenderness in the epigastric region. Serum amylase is 6000U/L. His WCC is 16,000/mm^3. His calcium level is low. An erect chest X-ray shows no gas under the diaphragm.

What is the most appropriate investigation in the management of this patient?

a. Abdominal ultrasound scan.
b. Serum lipase level.
c. Contrast-enhanced CT scan of the abdomen.
d. Endoscopic retrograde cholangiopancreatography.
e. Endoscopic ultrasound.

Q3
SBA

A 54-year-old female who is awaiting cholecystectomy for gallstones presents with constant severe upper abdominal pain of 1 day's duration. The abdomen is distended and there is tenderness in the epigastric region. Serum amylase is 2000U/L. An ultrasound scan shows multiple gallbladder stones, a dilated bile duct (11mm) and a possible stone at the lower end of the bile duct.

What is the most appropriate next step in the management of this patient?

a. Endoscopic retrograde cholangiogram, endoscopic sphincterotomy and stone extraction.
b. Emergency laparoscopic cholecystectomy.
c. Conservative management of acute pancreatitis.
d. Laparotomy, on-table cholangiogram and exploration of the bile duct.
e. Contrast-enhanced CT scan.

Q4
SBA

Which one of the following is unlikely to occur as a complication of gallstone pancreatitis?

a. Pancreatic necrosis.
b. Pancreatic duct disruption.
c. Pancreatic pleural effusion.
d. Pancreatic pseudocyst.
e. Pancreatic calcification.
f. Inflammatory pancreatic head mass.

Q5
True/False

a. Complete resolution occurs in the majority of patients with acute pancreatitis.
b. A systemic inflammatory response is responsible for multiple organ failure during the first week after the onset of acute pancreatitis.
c. Infected pancreatic necrosis is an indication for pancreatic necrosectomy.
d. Splenic vein thrombosis is a recognised complication of acute pancreatitis.
e. Urgent ERCP and an endoscopic sphincterotomy is indicated in patients with acute severe alcoholic pancreatitis.

Q6
True/False

Complications of acute pancreatitis include:

a. Acute fluid collections.
b. Portal vein thrombosis.
c. Intra-abdominal haemorrhage.
d. Pancreatic duct disruption.
e. Pleural effusion.

Q7
True/False

The following are considered as adverse prognostic criteria of acute severe pancreatitis.

a. Age above 55.
b. WCC more than 16,000/mm^3.
c. C-reactive protein more than 150mg/L.
d. Hypocalcaemia <2mmol/L.
e. Hypoxaemia <60mmHg.

Q8
True/False

Recurrent acute pancreatitis is recognised in patients with:

a. Pancreatic divism.
b. Gallstones.
c. Excessive alcohol consumption.
d. Primary hyperparathyroidism.
e. Peptic ulcer disease.

Answers overleaf

Self-assessment answers

Q1 1. (d), 2. (c), 3. (a), 4. (b).

Q2 (c).

Explanatory notes

This patient has acute alcoholic pancreatitis. He has had symptoms for 3 days. He is hypocalcaemic with a raised WCC. A contrast-enhanced CT scan is the best investigation to assess the extent of local pancreatic injury. Poor enhancement with contrast identifies early pancreatic necrosis. Because the initial clinical picture is suggestive of acute severe pancreatitis, the CT findings will also act as a baseline for comparison if he develops pancreatic necrosis.

Q3 (a). This is best practice based on BSG guidelines.

Q4 (e).

Explanatory notes

Pancreatic calcification is a hallmark of chronic pancreatitis. Chronic alcohol abuse is the most common cause of pancreatic calcification in the East. It is very rare for gallstones to cause chronic pancreatitis.

In the tropical and subtropical regions of the world, a condition referred to as tropical chronic calcific pancreatitis (TCCP) is increasingly recognised. TCCP is characterised by extensive pancreatic calcification in childhood, diabetes in adolescence and death in the prime of life.

Q5 a. (T), b. (T), c. (T), d. (T), e. (F).

Q6 a. (T), b. (T), c. (T), d. (T), f. (T).

Q7 a. (T), b. (T), c. (T), d. (T), e. (T).

Q8 a. (T), b. (T), c. (T), d. (T), e. (F).

Explanatory notes

Pancreatic divism is a condition where the main pancreatic duct drains via the minor papilla. Pancreatic divism is an embryological abnormality which results from defective fusion between the dorsal and ventral pancreatic buds. Some patients with pancreatic divism develop recurrent pancreatitis. The cause of pancreatitis is believed to be due to increased pancreatic ductal pressure because of the insufficient outlet at the minor papilla for the drainage of the main pancreatic duct.

A significant percentage of patients respond to widening of the minor papilla by endoscopic minor papilla sphincterotomy.

Chapter 7

Dyspepsia

Learning objectives

- To learn to evaluate patients presenting with dyspepsia.
- To learn the clinical presentation of patients with gastro-oesophageal reflux disease (GORD).
- To recollect the physiological mechanisms that prevent gastro-oesophageal reflux and the pathological processes that lead to GORD.
- To understand the diagnostic and therapeutic approach to a patient with suspected GORD.
- To learn the indications for surgery and the surgical options for GORD.

Case scenario

A 55-year-old female is referred with a 4-month history of epigastric pain, heartburn and regurgitation. Her symptoms are worse at night, after meals and when she lies down. She denies dysphagia or weight loss. Lately she has become reluctant to eat large meals because of the pain and abdominal distension after meals. She has a reasonable appetite. Since the onset of the symptoms she has had an intermittent early morning wheeze and some hoarseness in the morning. Her primary care physician has commenced her on omeprazole which she has taken for the previous 6 weeks and this treatment has partially resolved her symptoms.

She has no past medical problems. She is a non-smoker and consumes about a bottle of wine a week. She has had three children. She is not on any other medications except omeprazole. Her mother is known to have gallstones but has not had surgery for it.

Her primary care physician has obtained an ultrasound scan of her abdomen. This shows a solitary gallstone in a thin-walled gallbladder. She is moderately obese. No abnormalities are detected on examination.

The most likely clinical diagnosis: dyspepsia due to gastro-oesophageal reflux disease associated with silent aspiration and pharyngitis.

What is dyspepsia?

The SIGN guidelines refer to dyspepsia as "pain or discomfort in the upper abdomen usually in the form of indigestion".

In general the word dyspepsia is used by many clinicians to describe a collection of symptoms referable to the upper gastrointestinal tract. The symptoms are:

- Upper abdominal pain.
- Abdominal distension.
- Upper abdominal discomfort.
- Nausea with or without vomiting.
- Heartburn.
- Acid regurgitation.
- Abdominal distension after meals.
- Abdominal distension during the course of a normal meal (early satiety).

These symptoms may be intermittent or progressive. The severity of the symptoms may vary. In general such symptoms are very common. Many have experienced these symptoms at some stage of their life. But for some, the symptoms can be severe and disabling.

In approximately 50% of cases, a cause can be found for the dyspeptic symptoms. This is classified as organic dyspepsia. The commonest cause of organic dyspepsia is gastro-oesophageal reflux disease.

Other causes are:

- Peptic ulcer disease.
- Gallstone disease.
- Chronic pancreatitis.
- Oesophagogastric cancer.

However, in approximately 50%, a definitive diagnosis cannot be made after investigations for dyspepsia. This is classified as functional dyspepsia.

Some symptoms may dominate in patients with functional dyspepsia. Based on this, several subgroups of patients can be identified and grouped under functional dyspepsia. This approach is useful in order to formulate a treatment strategy. For example, if the dyspeptic symptoms are suggestive of peptic ulcer disease, such as epigastric pain related to meals, nocturnal pain and periodicity, and a peptic ulcer is not identified at endoscopy, then the condition is referred to as functional dyspepsia of ulcer type.

Heartburn and acid regurgitation are the cardinal symptoms of symptomatic gastro-oesophageal reflux. However, during investigations, if no objective evidence of reflux such as endoscopic changes, manometric evidence of low oesophageal sphincter pressure or evidence of reflux on 24-hour pH monitoring is found, these patients are classified as functional dyspepsia of reflux type.

It is also important to appreciate that in more than 50% patients with symptomatic gastro-oesophageal reflux, an endoscopic finding of oesophagitis is either minimal or absent.

Sometimes dyspeptic symptoms may be associated with longstanding colonic symptoms such as an increased frequency of stools, abdominal colic and a sense of incomplete evacuation of faeces especially in the morning. These symptoms are suggestive of irritable bowel syndrome (IBS). If no evidence of colon cancer, polyps and inflammatory bowel disease is found, these patients are classified as functional dyspepsia of IBS type. They may respond to antispasmodics.

Some patients with functional dyspepsia may not fit into any of the subgroups. They are classified in a group termed as functional dyspepsia of an indeterminate type.

What is the next step?

- This patient has recent onset progressive dyspepsia and clinical features suggestive of respiratory involvement due to gastro-oesophageal reflux. She has had a partial response to treatment with proton pump inhibitors (PPIs).
- She undergoes upper GI endoscopy.

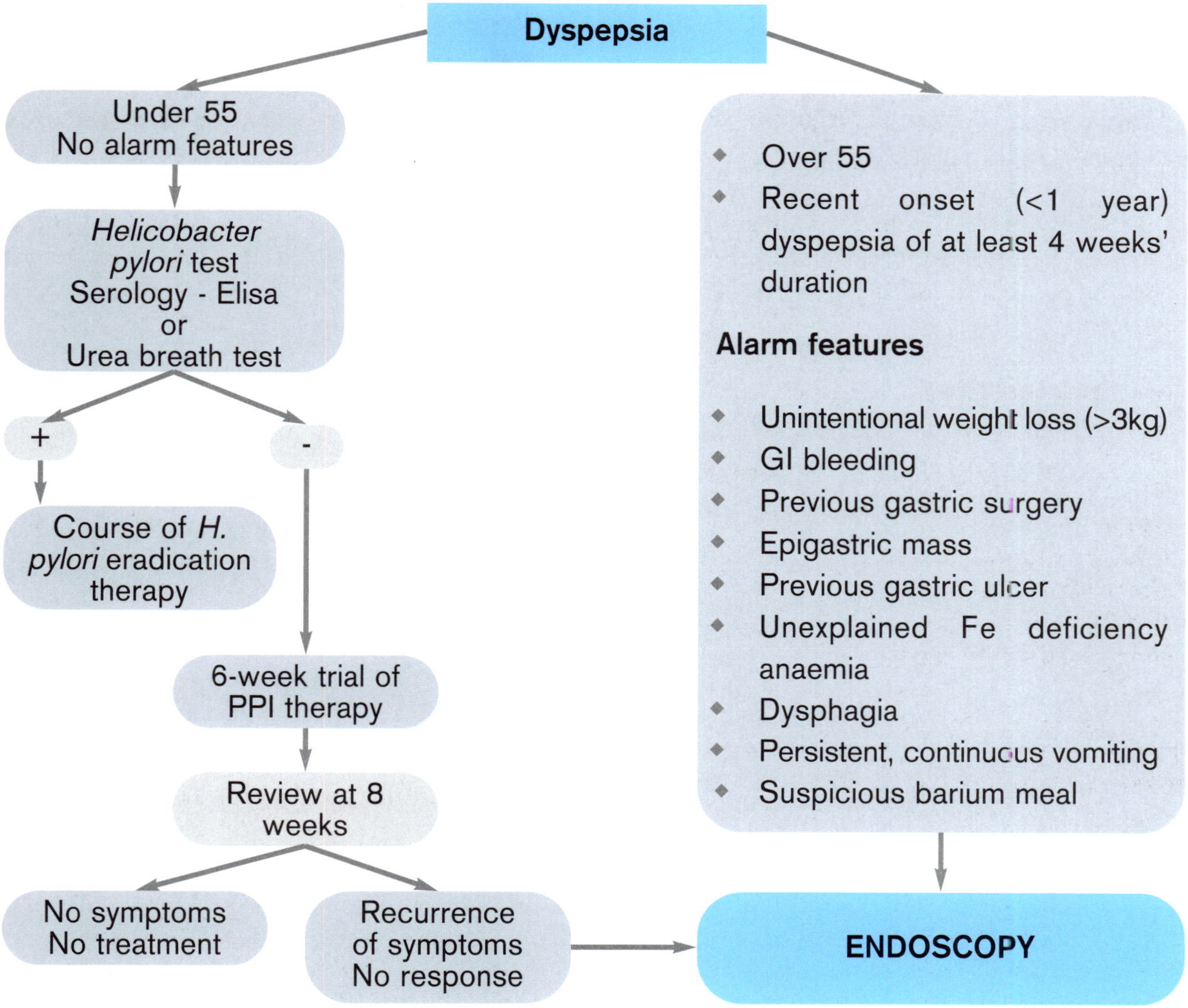

Figure 1. BSG guidelines for dyspepsia.

Progress of the patient

- The findings of the endoscopy are as follows:
  - small hiatus hernia;
  - moderate oesophagitis of the lower oesophagus;
  - stomach - mild patchy mucosal congestion;
  - duodenum - D1, D2 - normal;
  - the rapid urease test (CLO - Campylobacter-like organism test) is negative for *Helicobacter pylori*.
- Her haemoglobin is 14.9g/dL. She is not anaemic.

Should all patients with dyspepsia undergo upper GI endoscopy?

No. Based on the most recent BSG guidelines the clinical pathway given above is followed by many clinicians (Figure 1).

Progress of the patient

- The patient is informed that she has reflux of acidic gastric juice which has caused inflammation of the oesophagus.
- The wheezing episodes at night and the hoarseness she is experiencing is possibly related to episodes of silent aspiration she may be having especially at night.
- Because she has had a partial response to omeprazole she is advised to continue the same medication but at a higher dose of 40mg twice a day for a further 6 weeks.
- She is requested to report to the clinic in 8 weeks to assess the response.
- She is advised to lose weight, to sleep a little upright and to have small frequent meals. She is requested to avoid meals 2-3 hours prior to bedtime, to reduce the intake of fatty food and to reduce alcohol consumption.
- The fact that she is a non-smoker is helpful.

Clinical points

- Medical treatment with PPIs combined with lifestyle therapy is the initial treatment for GORD.
- High doses of PPIs may be required for severe symptoms or resistant oesophagitis.
- Patients with extra-oesophageal symptoms and pharyngeal reflux may be less responsive to medical treatment.
- Alternative diagnoses must be excluded in patients who do not respond to PPIs.

Progress of the patient

- The patient reports to the clinic 8 weeks later. She has had some improvement with omeprazole 40mg twice a day but had to reduce the dose again because she developed loose motions.
- Her disability is worse at night and the symptoms are precipitated by lying down.
- She wants to know whether her gallstone may be the cause of all these problems.
- She is concerned because her next door neighbour had complications from gallstones and had to undergo emergency surgery.
- She is advised that her clinical picture is suggestive of reflux of gastric contents into her oesophagus due to malfunctioning of the valve at the lower end of the gullet and is very unlikely to be due to gallstones.
- She is also advised that asymptomatic gallstones are not uncommon and surgery is not recommended for asymptomatic gallstones.
- She is reassured that, according to the present evidence, asymptomatic gallstones rarely cause problems and if a complication is to occur she will have some symptoms prior to it.
- She is referred for oesophageal manometry, 24-hour pH studies and a barium swallow and screening for objective assessment of her reflux.

Patients with chronic cholecystitis due to gallstones may present with dyspepsia and right hypochondrial pain. However, this patient's symptoms are not typical of gallstones. Her symptoms are typical of gastro-oesophageal reflux.

Moreover, her ultrasound scan has shown a thin-walled gallbladder and a solitary gallstone. If she had chronic cholecystitis, the usual finding would be a contracted or thick-walled gallbladder. She also has a familial predisposition to form gallstones. Therefore, it is very likely that she has asymptomatic gallstones.

Many studies have been done on the natural history of asymptomatic gallstones. These studies have confirmed that asymptomatic gallstones rarely cause problems and if a patient is to develop complications, it is usually preceded by the onset of some symptoms. Therefore, surgery is not advocated for asymptomatic gallstones. The slightly increased risk of carcinoma in longstanding gallstones is not considered as an indication for surgery. However, prophylactic cholecystectomy is indicated for patients with asymptomatic gallbladder stones in the endemic areas for gallbladder cancers (e.g. Chile).

Why do some patients with GORD not respond to medical therapy?

It is likely that she may belong to the subgroup of patients with significantly low pressures at the lower oesophageal sphincter due to the mechanical failure of the sphincter mechanism.

Normal physiological mechanisms are important in preventing reflux. Although there is no anatomical sphincter at the lower oesophagus the musculature acts like a physiological sphincter.

The lower oesophageal sphincter serves as a zone of increased pressure between the positive pressure in the stomach and the negative pressure in the chest.

Apart from the increased tone of the lower oesophageal musculature, certain anatomical factors such as the length of intra-abdominal oesophagus (which is exposed to a high intra-abdominal pressure), the crural diaphragm which is attached to the oesophagus by the phreno-oesophageal ligament and the acute angle at the cardio-oesophageal junction (angle of His) contribute to prevent reflux.

A widened oesophageal hiatus can lead to migration of the cardio-oesophageal sphincter with part of the stomach moving up into the chest. This anatomical abnormality is called a hiatus hernia. A hiatus hernia is a very common finding in the middle-aged and elderly. The majority are asymptomatic. However, in some, because the lower oesophageal sphincter is abnormally located in the chest, the anti-reflux mechanism may be compromised.

In health the lower oesophageal sphincter is closed most of the time. It opens in response to a food bolus when the bolus reaches the lower oesophagus. A certain amount of reflux is possible when the lower oesophageal sphincter opens to create the way for the oncoming food bolus, but a pool of alkaline saliva which comes with the food will take care of it by 'washing off' the transient acid bath of the lower oesophagus.

The lower oesophageal sphincter opens up from time to time, independent of swallowing. These episodes of sphincter relaxation are called transient lower oesophageal sphincter relaxation (TLOSR). TLOSR is shown to occur more frequently in patients with symptomatic gastro-oesophageal reflux.

Abnormalities of any of the anatomical or physiological mechanisms can contribute to abnormal reflux.

Progress of the patient

- Manometry identifies a low oesophageal sphincter pressure which is compatible with incompetent sphincter activity.
- The 24-hour pH study confirms significant reflux which correlates with the clinical episodes of reflux pain.
- The barium swallow confirms a hiatus hernia.
- She is offered surgical therapy and decides to undergo a laparoscopic Nissen fundoplication.

The objective evidence is that there is lower oesophageal sphincter dysfunction in this patient. She has not responded well to high-dose PPIs. She could not tolerate an 8-week course of PPIs because of the side effects. Her reflux symptoms are disabling. There is clear justification to offer her surgery.

The majority of patients with GORD respond to PPIs and lifestyle therapy. They can be managed with intermittent treatment during relapses. It is not uncommon for GORD to relapse. A relapse is not an indication for surgery because the majority respond to intermittent treatment. This means that a patient is given a 6-8 week course of PPIs. Some may wish to be on long-term treatment with PPIs at a smaller dose. Some patients are offered on demand therapy which means taking a dose of PPIs whenever the patient has symptoms. These are the different approaches practised by primary care physicians, once a sinister lesion is ruled out.

The NICE guidelines (2005) recommend that patients who are on treatment for dyspepsia should be encouraged to try stepping down or to stop treatment. A return to self-treatment with antacids is considered appropriate.

The standard work-up prior to surgical therapy for GORD are:

- Endoscopy.
- Manometry.
- 24-hour pH probe testing.
- Barium swallow and screening.

Not all surgeons routinely perform all four procedures.

Upper GI endoscopy

Upper GI endoscopy evaluates the severity of the oesophagitis (Figure 2). However, there is a poor correlation between the pathological changes and the severity of symptoms. The endoscopy will also be able to demonstrate the presence of Barrett's mucosa (see Chapter 9) and provides an opportunity for biopsies to exclude *Helicobacter pylori* infection, oesophagogastric cancer and peptic ulcer disease. The presence of a hiatus hernia may be noted.

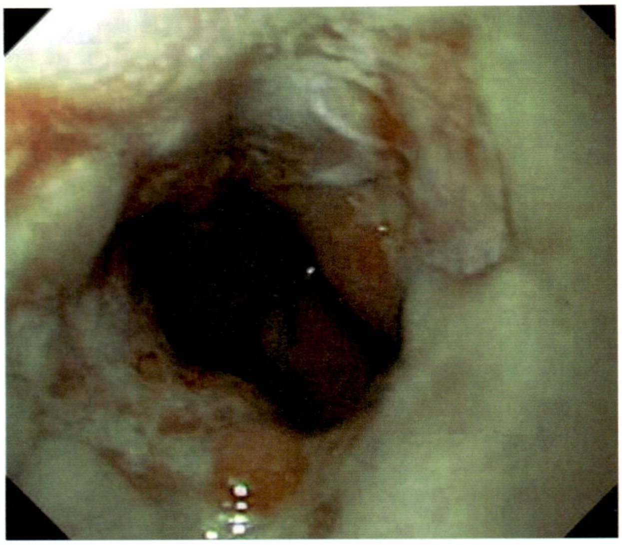

Figure 2. Endoscopic view of oesophagitis. ***Reproduced with permission from Hans Bjorknas, Gastrolab, Finland. www.gastrolab.net.***

Manometry

This test evaluates the competency of the lower oesophageal sphincter. It also helps to recognise other motility disorders such as achalasia of the cardia and diffuse oesophageal spasm.

24-hour pH studies

24-hour pH studies help to quantify the reflux severity and correlate symptoms with the reflux episodes.

Barium swallow and screening

A barium swallow and screening helps to identify the location of the cardio-oesophageal junction in relation to the diaphragm, identifies the hiatus hernia and also demonstrates spontaneous reflux.

Surgery is indicated in patients with documented GORD who have persistent symptoms while taking a maximum dose of PPIs, those who are intolerant to PPIs or those who do not wish to continue with life-long medications.

The operation commonly performed is the Nissen fundoplication. This can be performed by open surgery or by the laparoscopic approach. With the advent of the laparoscopic approach and the advancement of technology to assess the lower oesophageal sphincter mechanism objectively, more patients are opting for a laparoscopic Nissen fundoplication.

What is a Nissen fundoplication?

In a Nissen fundoplication, the lower oesophagus and fundus of the stomach are mobilised and the fundus of the stomach is 'wrapped around' the lower oesophagus to create a valve effect. What is commonly performed is the 360° wrap. Some surgeons prefer partial fundoplication. Due to its minimal invasiveness, the laparoscopic approach has become more popular over the open approach.

In many series the long-term success of fundoplication exceeds 90%.

There is a small (0.1-0.5%) but important postoperative mortality associated with anti-reflux surgery (NICE 2005).

Postoperative problems of Nissen fundoplication include delay in intestinal function causing bloating, gagging and vomiting. These side effects usually resolve in a few weeks. Other complications are:

- An excessively wrapped fundus which causes dysphagia.
- Wound infection.
- Injury to nearby organs.
- Muscle spasms after swallowing food.

The muscle spasms can cause intense pain and patients may require a liquid diet sometimes for weeks. This is rare but it can occur more frequently in children with neurologic abnormalities.

Long-term failure rates of 29% have been reported after fundoplication. Hiatal herniation is the most common reason for surgical failure and the need for a repeat fundoplication. With increasing experience and better selection criteria improved long-term results have been reported in newer trials. There is evidence that re-do surgery may produce satisfactory results.

Endoscopic techniques are being developed to increase the lower oesophageal sphincter pressure to prevent reflux. One such technique is trans-oral flexible endoscopic suturing (Bard s procedure) which uses a tiny device at the end of the endoscope that acts like a miniature sewing machine. It places stitches in two locations near the lower oesophageal sphincter, which are then tied to tighten the valve and increase pressure. There is no incision and no need

Progress of the patient

- During the first clinic visit at 4 weeks she reports a marked reduction in heartburn. She also complains of having a sensation of a lump in the back of the chest bone, some pain in the lower chest area which radiates upwards, abdominal fullness and some upper abdominal pain after meals. The symptoms are worse on standing and better when lying down. She has no dysphagia.
- The surgeon explains that a small percentage of patients may experience a sensation of a lump behind the sternum, fullness, bloating, and sometimes upper abdominal pain due to the inability to belch as a result of the fundal wrap. This is called gas bloat syndrome. If the wrap is too tight she will have dysphagia. In the upright position, air in the stomach moves to the upper parts of the stomach causing bloating, fullness and an urge to belch. Because she cannot belch after the fundoplication, the sensation persists. The severity and duration of discomfort varies among patients. It is impossible to predict the duration of the symptoms but in the majority these symptoms subside.
- The patient states that she is happy to live with these symptoms rather than the disabling heartburn. She has already stopped omeprazole on her own. She is relieved to hear that these symptoms too wil resolve with time.

for general anaesthesia. However, according to NICE guidelines (IPG 115, 2005), the evidence for efficiency is not adequate for this procedure to be used without special arrangements for consent and for audit and research.

Suggested reading

1. Britiish Society of Gastroenterology. Dyspepsia management guidelines. BSG, 2002.
2. Scottish Intercollegiate Guidelines Network. Dyspepsia: national clinical guideline, SIGN 2003; 68.
3. McSherry CK, Ferstenberg H, Calhoun WF, Lahman E, Virshup M. The natural history of diagnosed gallstone disease in symptomatic and asymptomatic patients. *Ann Surg* 1985; 202(1): 59-63.
4. National Institute for Health and Clinical Excellence. Dyspepsia: management of dyspepsia in adults in primary care. NICE, 2005.
5. DeVault KR, Castell DO. Updated guidelines for the diagnosis and treatment of gastroesophageal reflux disease. *Am J Gastroenterol* 2005; 100(1): 190-200.
6. Sandbu R, Khamis H, Gustavsson S, Haglund U. Long-term results of antireflux surgery indicate the need for a randomized clinical trial. *Br J Surg* 2002; 89(2): 225-30.
7. Oelschlager BK, Quiroga E, Parra JD, Cahill M, Polissar N, Pellegrini CA. Long-term outcomes after laparoscopic antireflux surgery. *Am J Gastroenterol* 2008; 103(2): 280-7.
8. National Institute for Health and Clinical Excellence. Endoluminal gastroplication for gastro-oesophageal reflux Disease. NICE, 2005.

Self-assessment

Q1
EMQ

a. 6-week course of omeprazole.
b. *Helicobacter pylori* testing and a 6-week trial of omeprazole.
c. Change the medication to esomeprazole.
d. Consider laparoscopic Nissen fundoplication.
e. Add antacid therapy to omeprazole.
f. *Helicobacter pylori* eradication treatment as empirical therapy.

Select the most appropriate protocol from above for the case scenarios described below.

1. A 35-year-old female presents with a 1-month history of epigastric pain, heartburn and regurgitation. The symptoms are worse at night, after meals and on lying down. She has no dysphagia, weight loss or loss of appetite.
2. A 68-year-old male with chronic obstructive pulmonary disease (COPD) due to heavy smoking presents with a 3-month history of heartburn and regurgitation. He has had partial relief with ranitidine. He has no ischaemic heart disease. Upper GI endoscopy shows mild oesophagitis and a negative CLO test.
3. A 35-year-old bank executive who is on the maximum dose of omeprazole for longstanding GORD presents with decreasing libido which he attributes to omeprazole. He tends to miss taking his medications at times due to the pressure of work. His symptoms at times are disabling.

Q2
EMQ

a. Peptic ulcer disease.
b. Gallstone disease.
c. Chronic pancreatitis.
d. Gastric carcinoma.
e. Antral gastritis.
f. Cancer of the pancreas.

Select the most likely clinical diagnosis from the conditions mentioned above for the case scenarios described below.

1. An elderly male presents with anaemia, weight loss, severe loss of appetite and recent onset dysphagia.
2. An elderly male presents with weight loss, dyspepsia and recent onset jaundice with pale stools. He has a palpable gallbladder.
3. Longstanding recurrent epigastric pain after meals, periodicity and nocturnal pain.
4. An obese female with recurrent right hypochondrial pain and nausea.

Q3
SBA

Which of the following conditions is considered as the commonest cause of organic dyspepsia?

a. Peptic ulcer disease.
b. Chronic cholecystitis.
c. Gastro-oesophageal reflux disease.
d. Gastric carcinoma.
e. Chronic pancreatitis.

Q4
True/False

a. Reflux of gastric contents to the lower oesophagus occurs independently of swallowing.
b. Gastro-oesophageal reflux disease does not occur in the absence of hiatus hernia.
c. Symptoms of gastro-oesophageal reflux could occur in the absence of oesophagitis.
d. Gasto-oesophageal reflux predisposes to Barrett's oesophagus.
e. The majority of patients with gastro-oesophageal reflux disease respond to medical treatment.

Answers overleaf

Self-assessment answers

Q1 1. (b), 2. (a), 3. (d).

Explanatory notes

1. A young female with a short history with no alarming features. This is a very common presentation in primary care. *Helicobacter pylori* testing with a urea breath test or serology and a 6-week trial of omeprazole is in order, based on the guidelines.

2. Reflux is not uncommon in COPD. Proton pump inhibitors (e.g. omeprazole) are shown to be superior to H2 receptor antagonists (e.g. ranitidine) for GORD. He has no *Helicobacter pylori* infection. Change to a PPI would be the most appropriate next step.

3. A young man with a stressful lifestyle. He is on the maximum dose of medication with possible side effects. He has a problem with compliance. The next step is to consider surgery.

Q2 1. (d), 2. (f), 3. (a), 4. (b).

Explanatory notes

1. Anaemia, loss of appetite and dysphagia in an elderly male is highly suggestive of a gastric cancer obstructing the gastric inlet.

2. Painless jaundice, weight loss and a palpable gallbladder in an elderly male is highly suspicious of a malignant process obstructing the bile duct below the insertion of the cystic duct. Pancreatic head cancer involves the intrapancreatic portion of the bile duct and causes obstructive jaundice. This is explained in Courvoisier's law (see Chapter 5).

3. Epigastric pain related to meals, periodicity and nocturnal pain are characteristic features of chronic duodenal ulceration.

4. A fat forty flatulent fertile female is the classical patient with gallbladder dyspepsia. The pathological process is chronic cholecystitis.

Q3 (c).

Q4 a. (T), b. (F), c. (T), d. (T), e. (T).

Explanatory notes

c. In more than 50% of patients with symptomatic gastro-oesophageal reflux, endoscopic findings of oesophagitis are either minimal or absent. This is an important point because patients may be at a loss to understand why the endoscopy result is normal in the presence of symptoms.

These patients may have microscopic oesophagitis or the lower oesophageal mucosa may be hypersensitive to acid. Some gastroenterologists routinely biopsy the lower oesophageal mucosa in all patients with symptomatic gastro-oesophageal reflux even in the absence of endoscopic changes.

Chapter 8

Acute upper gastrointestinal haemorrhage

Learning objectives

- To be familiar with the common causes of acute upper GI haemorrhage.
- To learn the natural course and adverse prognostic factors.
- To understand the importance of the initial evaluation and be able to recognise the severity of blood loss in acute haemorrhage.
- To be able to outline the resuscitation and treatment strategies for patients presenting with acute upper GI haemorrhage and shock.

Case scenario

A 54-year-old male presents with tarry-coloured stools and a feeling of light-headedness. During the last 24 hours he has had several bowel movements containing tarry-coloured stools and he has fainted once. During the last year or so he has been frequently troubled with back pain and has been on ibuprofen for the last 8 months. He gives no history of altered bowels, similar episodes of tarry stools or bleeding per rectum. He consumes 2-3 pints of beer during weekends. He denies smoking.

On examination, he is pale. He looks lethargic but conscious and co-operative. His temperature is 37°C, pulse rate is 120/minute and BP measured in the supine position is 90/70mm Hg. The abdomen is mildly distended. Slight tenderness is elicited in the epigastrium. Rectal examination reveals black stools but no masses are felt.

The most likely clinical diagnosis: Class III haemorrhage due to a bleeding peptic ulcer or gastric erosions caused by ibuprofen (a non-steroidal anti-inflammatory drug).

What is the next step?

- Urgent fluid resuscitation with 2 x 14G cannulae to the antecubital fossae and 1L of N saline to each arm, after collecting blood for cross-matching.
- Emergency cross-matching of 5 units of blood.
- An FBC and a coagulation, liver and renal profile are requested.
- Catheter and hourly monitoring of urine output.
- Close monitoring of the pulse rate, blood pressure and severity of malaena stool.
- Omeprazole 80mg IV bolus injection (as empirical therapy due to history of non-steroidal anti-inflammatory drug [NSAID] treatment).

What is a Class III haemorrhage?

Acute haemorrhage from any cause is classified into four classes, according to the Advanced Trauma Life Support course® (ATLS®) of the American College of Surgeons (Table 1).

This patient's systolic blood pressure in the supine position is 90mm Hg. Therefore, his blood pressure in the upright position must be lower than 90mmHg. He has a Class III haemorrhage.

The BSG's guidelines and other guidelines recommend categorising patients with acute upper GI haemorrhage at the time of admission into low or high risk of death.

In practice the two criteria to assess the risk of death are:

- Severity of the bleeding episode.
- Associated comorbidities.

The Rockall scoring system for the risk of re-bleeding and death after admission to hospital for acute gastrointestinal bleeding is based on the following independent risk factors:

- Increasing age. There is a close relationship between mortality and age. The older the patient, the higher the risk of death.
- Comorbidity. The number and severity of comorbid illnesses are closely related to mortality. Patients who have advanced renal and liver disease, and disseminated cancer have the worst outcomes.
- Shock. Defined as a pulse rate of more than 100 beats/minute and systolic blood pressure of less than 100mm Hg.
- Endoscopic findings.
  High risk:
  - spurting vessel;
  - oozing vessel;
  - visible vessel at the base of the ulcer;
  - adherent blood clot on the ulcer.

Table 1. Classification of acute haemorrhage.

Class I (in adults of 70Kg weight)

Loss of up to 15% of circulating blood volume (up to 750ml loss).

- Usually no physical signs.

Class II

Loss of up to 30% of circulating blood volume (up to 1500ml).

- Tachycardia.
- Reduced pulse pressure (due to peripheral vasoconstriction causing increase in the diastolic pressure).
- Normal systolic blood pressure.

Class III

Loss of up to 30-40% of circulating blood volume (up to 2000ml).

- Persistent drop of systolic blood pressure.

Class IV

Loss of more than 40% of circulating volume.

- The patient has catastrophic haemorrhage.

Low risk:
- ulcer with a clean base;
- Mallory-Weiss tear.

Because most scoring systems depend on endoscopic findings, no scoring system will accurately predict the risk of death at the initial assessment. Therefore, the definition of risk remains a matter of clinical judgement. However, at the initial assessment most clinicians classify patients into two groups: mild/moderate risk or high risk.

Mild or moderate risk:

- Normal pulse and blood pressure.
- Haemoglobin concentration is greater than 10g/dL.
- No significant comorbidities.
- Age less than 60 years.

Management plan:

- Admission to the ward.
- Hourly measurement of pulse rate, blood pressure and urine output.
- Endoscopy is undertaken on the next available list.

High risk:

- Age above 60 years.
- Pulse greater than 100 beats/minute.
- Systolic blood pressure less than 100mm Hg.
- Haemoglobin less than 10g/dL.
- Significant comorbid factors.

Management plan:

- Initial resuscitation.
- Close monitoring in the HDU setting.
- Central venous pressure (CVP) monitoring may be needed in patients with ischaemic heart disease or heart failure.
- IV omeprazole.
- Urgent upper GI endoscopy.
- A general anaesthetic and ventilation may be needed for endoscopy, if there is evidence of hypoxaemia.

Clinical points

- A critical aspect of the initial evaluation is the assessment of the severity of blood loss and comorbid factors.
- Prompt attention to airway, breathing and circulation is mandatory.
- Patients who are agitated or have impaired respiratory status must have endotracheal intubation and resuscitation prior to endoscopy.
- The sequence of management of acute upper GI haemorrhage must be in the following order:
  - resuscitation;
  - diagnosis - the cause of bleeding;
  - treatment.

What is the rationale for giving a bolus dose of IV omeprazole to this patient?

Clot formation over the arteries is pH-dependent and a gastric pH above 6 is thought to be critical for platelet aggregation. In clinical practice many gastroenterologists would initiate treatment with PPIs prior to endoscopy.

The adjuvant use of high-dose PPIs in endoscopic therapy has been endorsed in consensus statements and confirmed by meta-analyses.

Progress of the patient

- The patient is monitored in the HDU. The patient's pulse rate decreases to 100/minute and blood pressure stabilises at 100/70mm Hg after infusion of 2L of N saline and 2 units of blood.
- Results of investigations:
  - Hb 10g/dL;
  - INR 1.2;
  - liver profile - normal;
  - renal profile - normal.

Progress of the patient

- CVP monitoring is considered but not performed as the parameters are stable. The patient is scheduled for an upper GI endoscopy.
- After resuscitation to optimise the haemodynamic status, the patient is prepared for endoscopy to identify the source of bleeding.

In general, the causes of acute upper GI haemorrhage can be classified as variceal and non-variceal. Non-variceal causes are acute gastric erosions, peptic ulceration, oesophageal ulcers, Mallory-Weiss tears, gastric cancers and Dieulafoy's lesions.

A Mallory-Weiss tear is a linear mucosal tear in the lower oesophagus as a result of forceful vomiting or retching. The initial description was associated with alcoholic binge drinking. Although the initial bleeding may be heavy, in the majority the bleeding ceases without the need for active intervention.

A Dieulafoy's lesion (Dieulafoy is a French surgeon) is an uncommon cause of gastrointestinal bleeding in which significant, recurrent haemorrhage occurs from a pinpoint non-ulcerated arterial lesion, usually high in the gastric fundus.

Progress of the patient

- An upper GI endoscopy is performed. A 2cm chronic benign-looking duodenal ulcer is noted with a vessel at the base with some oozing. There is altered blood in the stomach. No oesophageal or gastric varices are seen.
- 1:10,000 epinephrine is injected around the ulcer and a heat probe is applied to the vessel to achieve haemostasis.
- An antral biopsy is done for the CLO test - *Helicobacter pylori* - negative.
- No biopsies from the ulcer are performed.
- An omeprazole 8mg hourly infusion is continued for 24 hours.
- The patient is monitored for re-bleeding.
- The patient responds to treatment.
- A soft diet is commenced by the second day.
- The patient is discharged on omeprazole 40mg daily to be reviewed in the clinic in 4 weeks.

Duodenal ulcers almost never become malignant. Therefore, biopsies are not done to assess malignancy. Some clinicians would obtain duodenal biopsies to assess *Helicobacter pylori* (HP) status. The highest density of HP has been shown to be in the gastric antrum and therefore the best site to obtain a biopsy for HP is a non-ulcerated area of the antrum.

What methods are available for endoscopic haemostasis?

This will depend on the cause of the bleeding. The common causes are chronic peptic ulcer disease, acute gastric erosions and oesophageal varices. Heavy bleeding form gastric cancers are uncommon.

Oesophageal varices

Banding and injection sclerotherapy are common endoscopic techniques used to control oesophageal varices. There is evidence that the results of banding are superior to injection scelerotherapy. If there is extensive bleeding from varices, balloon tamponade using a Sengstaken-Blakemore tube is attempted as the first resort. The objective is to gain control of haemorrhage and to establish a dry field for subsequent endotherapy. Balloon tamponade is used for 24-48 hours.

There is evidence that the use of systemic vasoconstrictor drugs such as vasopressin or its synthetic analogue, glypressin, is useful. Somatostatin or its synthetic analogue, octreotide, is also recommended. Endoscopy and banding are attempted after 24-48 hours. If bleeding continues a transjugular intrahepatic portosystemic shunt (TIPS) is the next option. Heavy bleeding and significant hepatic decompensation is associated with a high mortality.

Gastric varices may cause troublesome bleeding. They are less common than oesophageal varices. The incidence of bleeding is less than for oesophageal varices. The treatment of choice for gastric varices is cyanoacrylate glue. Cyanoacrylate glue becomes solidified within seconds when it comes into contact with biological tissue.

Peptic ulcers (Figures 1 and 2)

A range of endoscopic treatments are available to treat patients who have stigmata of recent haemorrhage. A meta-analysis of trials showed that endoscopic therapy reduces re-bleeding, the need for surgical intervention and mortality.

Endoscopic therapies include injections, and the application of heat or mechanical clips.

Injection

1:10,000 adrenaline solution in normal saline is injected around the bleeding point and then into the bleeding vessel. This approach will achieve primary haemostasis in up to 95% of patients, although bleeding will recur in 15-20%.

Application of heat

Thermal haemostasis is achieved using either a heater probe or multipolar coagulation. The heater probe includes a powerful water jet which aids removal of the overlying blood clot.

Argon plasma coagulation has also been shown to be effective for ulcer bleeding.

Mechanical clips

Mechanical clips can be applied to bleeding points and are particularly useful for actively bleeding large vessels.

Indications for repeat endoscopy

Repeat endoscopy is indicated:

- If there is clinical evidence of active re-bleeding suggested by the passage of fresh melaena or haematemesis, a fall in blood pressure, a rise in pulse rate, or a fall in central venous pressure.
- If there are concerns regarding the adequacy of the initial endoscopic therapy.

Indications for surgery

Active non-variceal gastrointestinal haemorrhage that cannot be stopped by endotherapy is an indication for surgery.

Follow-up of chronic peptic ulcers

During follow-up of chronic peptic ulcers:

- PPIs should be prescribed where applicable.
- Helicobacter should be eradicated if a positive test is found.

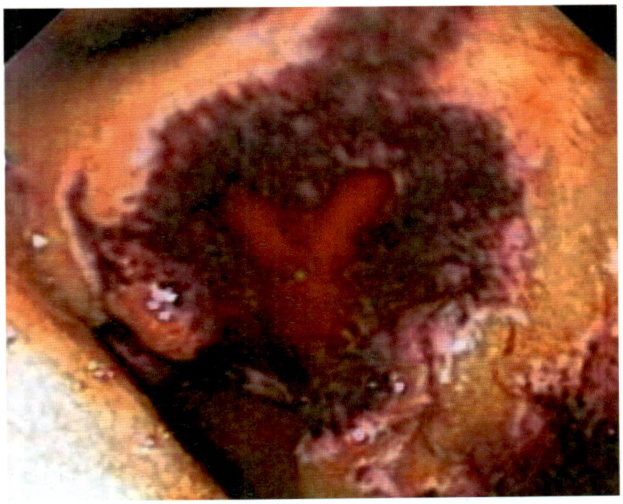

Figure 1. Chronic duodenal ulcer with evidence of bleeding. ***Reproduced with permission from Hans Bjorknas, Gastrolab, Finland. www.gastrolab.net.***

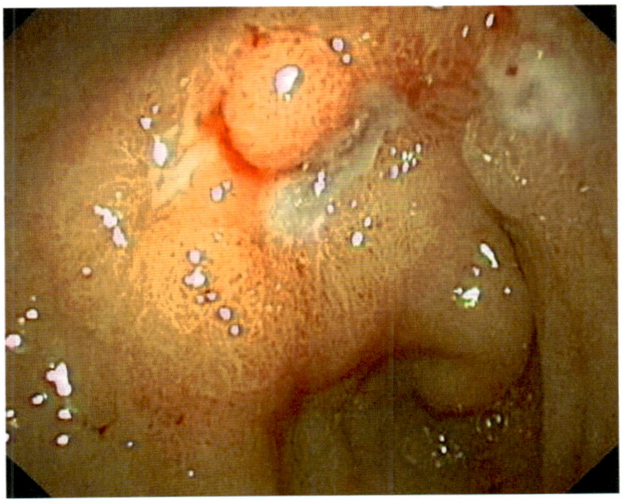

Figure 2. Chronic gastric ulcer with a visible vessel at the base. ***Reproduced with permission from Hans Bjorknas, Gastrolab, Finland. www.gastrolab.net.***

- Non-steroidal anti-inflammatory drugs or aspirin should be stopped.
- If the lesion is a gastric ulcer, it should be biopsied and, if negative, the endoscopy should be performed after 6 weeks to confirm ulcer healing and to exclude malignancy.
- Patients on steroids should be closely monitored and a PPI taken in conjunction with the steroid medication.

There is evidence that eradication of *Helicobacter pylori* in patients with a positive HP test cures peptic ulcer disease.

An algorithm for the management of acute upper GI haemorrhage is shown in Figure 3.

Progress of the patient

- At the follow-up clinic at 4 weeks the patient reports having no further episodes of haematemesis or melaena. The patient is on omeprazole 40mg/day. The endoscopy is repeated at 8 weeks, which shows that the ulcer has almost completely healed. The patient is advised to continue omeprazole at a reduced dose for a further 4 weeks. Because the CLO test is negative anti-*Helicobacter pylori* therapy is not given.

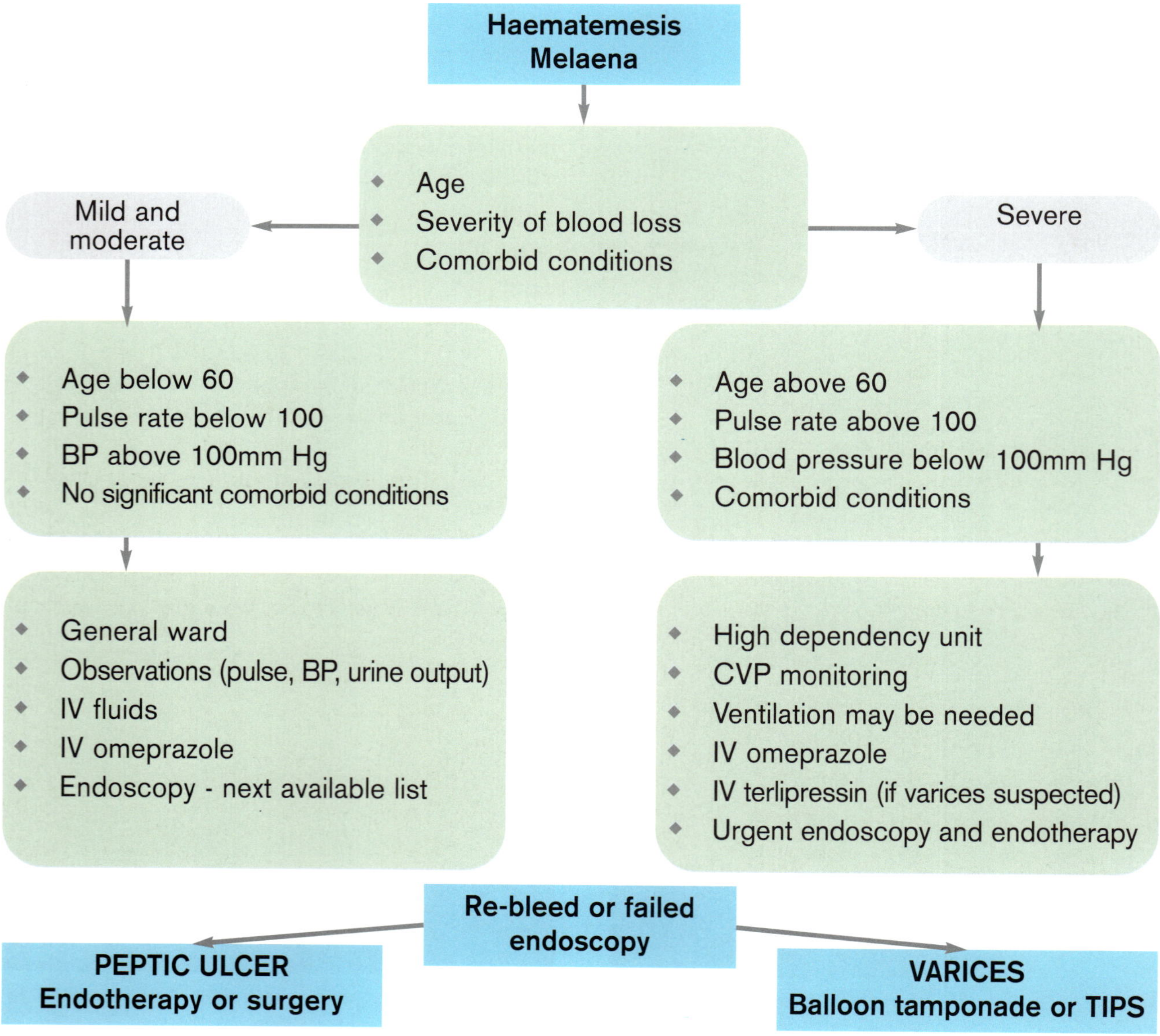

Figure 3. Algorithm for the management of acute upper GI haemorrhage.

Suggested reading

1. Palmer KR. Non-variceal upper gastrointestinal haemorrhage: guidelines. British Society of Gastroenterology Endoscopy Committee. *Gut* 2002; 51: 1-6
2. Rockall TA, Logan RFA, Devlin HB, *et al.* Incidence of and mortality from acute upper gastrointestinal haemorrhage in the United Kingdom. *BMJ* 1995; 311: 222-6.
3. Lau JY, Leung WK, Wu JCY, Chan FKL, *et al.* Omeprazole before endoscopy in patients with gastrointestinal bleeding. *New Engl J Med* 2007; 356: 1631-40.

Self-assessment

Q1
EMQ

a. Endoscopy on the next list.
b. Urgent endoscopy under sedation.
c. Treat with PPIs and arrange an outpatient endoscopy.
d. Emergency laparotomy.
e. Urgent endoscopy under general anaesthesia.

Given below are case scenarios of patients presenting with melaena. All had initial resuscitation with IV fluids, blood and IV omeprazole.

Select the most appropriate next step from the options given above for the case scenarios described below. One option can be selected only once.

1. A 54-year-old male who is on long-term ibuprofen. He is pale, agitated, with a pulse rate of 120/minute, BP of 90/70mm Hg and RR of 32/minute. Oxygen saturation on the pulse oximeter is 84%.
2. A 40-year-old non-alcoholic male, who is conscious, co-operative, pale, with a pulse rate of 86/minute, BP of 130/80mm Hg and RR of 20/minute.
3. A 65-year-old female on long-term NSAID therapy. She is pale, with a pulse rate of 110/minute, BP of 100/60mm Hg and RR of 22/minute.

Q2
EMQ

a. Cyanoacrylate glue injection.
b. Banding.
c. Heat probe.
d. Haemoclips.
e. 1 in 10,000 adrenaline infiltration.
f. Transjugular intrahepatic portosystemic shunt.

Select the treatment options which could be used to control haemorrhage for the conditions mentioned below. You may select one, more than one option or none for each condition.

1. Chronic duodenal ulcer.
2. Gastic varices.
3. Chronic benign gastric ulcer.
4. Oesophageal varices.

Q3
SBA

The surgical registrar is called at 8am to a medical ward to assess a patient who has presented with haematemesis and melaena the previous night. The observation chart indicates the following readings:

- Pulse rate: on admission (night) 120/minute, morning 130/minute.
- BP: on admission (night) 100/60mm Hg, morning 90/70mm Hg.

The patient has been transfused with two units of blood during the night.

What is the most appropriate clinical judgement?

a. Bleeding has ceased.
b. Class I haemorrhage.
c. Class II haemorrhage.
d. Class III haemorrhage.
e. Class IV haemorrhage.

Q4
True/False

The following statements are true/false with regard to haematemesis and melaena:

a. The number of comorbid illnesses are closely related to mortality.
b. Patients with massive haematemesis due to oesophageal varices must undergo banding of varices immediately.
c. Endoscopy must be performed under general anaesthesia in patients with impaired respiratory status.
d. A bolus dose of intravenous omeprazole is given prior to endoscopy.
e. Endoscopic treatment will achieve immediate control of bleeding in the majority with bleeding peptic ulcers.

Answers overleaf

Self-assessment answers

Q1 1. (e), 2. (a), 3. (b).

Q2 1. (c, d, e), 2. (a), 3. (c, d, e), 4. (b, f).

Q3 (c).

Q4 a. (T), b. (F), c. (T), d. (T), e. (T).

Chapter 9

Dysphagia

Learning objectives

- To recollect the clinical picture of a patient with malignant obstruction of the oesophagus and oesophagogastric junction.
- To learn the investigative modalities available and to understand how such information is used in pre-operative staging.
- To learn the pathophysiology and controversies in the management of Barrett's oesophagus.
- To appreciate the method of selection of patients for surgical consideration and the advantages and limitations of surgery.
- To learn the anatomical and pathological basis, and the outcome of surgery for oesophageal cancer.

Case scenario

A 65-year-old ex-sailor presents with dysphagia of 3 weeks' duration. He has a good appetite but finds it difficult to swallow, especially solid foods. He points to the mid-sternal area as the site of obstruction. He has been on antacids intermittently for heartburn and acid regurgitation for years.

He has no past history of ingestion of corrosive substances. He has smoked about 10 cigarettes a day for the last 10 years. He has no other significant comorbidities.

On examination he is obese. He is not pale. The chest, cardiovascular and abdominal examinations are normal.

The most likely clinical diagnosis: malignant obstruction of the oesophagus or gastric inlet.

The male sex, age above 60 and a history of smoking are the risk factors for oesophageal carcinoma in this patient. The longstanding reflux symptoms bring benign oesophageal stricture into the differential diagnosis. However, the working clinical diagnosis of this patient is a cancerous obstruction of the oesophagus or oesophagogastric junction.

Men are more likely to develop squamous carcinoma of the oesophagus. Tobacco smoking increases the risk of squamous carcinoma of the oesophagus by nine-fold. Longstanding symptomatic GORD is a recognised risk factor for Barrett's oesophagus and oesophageal adenocarcinoma.

In the last few decades the incidence of oesophageal and gastric cardia adenocarcinoma in both men and women has increased rapidly in the western world. The incidence of adenocarcinoma has overtaken squamous carcinoma at this level of the oesophagus. As well as the previously described risk factors (GORD, smoking), the increasing prevalence of obesity in the western world is recognised as an important factor responsible for this shift.

What is the next step?

- The patient has an upper gastrointestinal endoscopy (Figure 1).
- Endoscopy reveals an ulcerated growth extending from 38-40cm up to the cardio-oesophageal junction but not extending into the stomach. The tumour involves approximately 50% of the circumference. The remaining oesophagus, stomach and duodenum are normal.
- A total of five biopsies are obtained from the edge of the ulcer and a photograph is taken.
- As the ulcer appears to be malignant, a contrast CT scan of the thorax, abdomen and pelvis with intravenous contrast and gastric distension with oral contrast is performed.

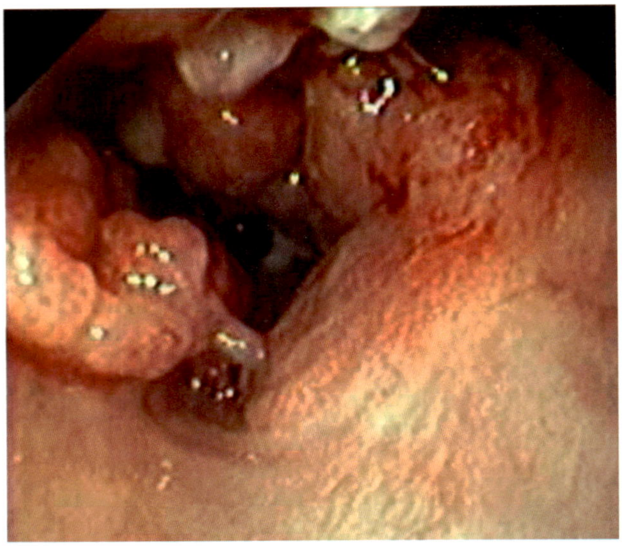

Figure 1. Endoscopic appearance of an oesophageal cancer. *Reproduced with permission from Hans Bjorknas, Gastrolab, Finland. www.gastrolab.net.*

Progress of the patient

- The CT and histology results are discussed at the MDT meeting.
- Histology confirms an adenocarcinoma in the setting of Barrett's oesophagus.
- A CT scan confirms an oesophageal tumour with no evidence of mediastinal, supraclavicular node and abdominal involvement. The liver and lungs are clear.
- As there is potential for a curative resection, the patient has an endoscopic ultrasound (EUS) scan for tumour staging.
- EUS demonstrates the tumour at 37-40cm, in the right lateral wall of the oesophagus extending from the 6 o'clock to 12 o'clock position, with a maximum thickness of 13mm, infiltrating the muscularis propria at 39cm. No nodes were identified. It is classified as a T2 tumour (Table 1).
- Because the tumour is at the cardio-oesophageal junction, and is an adenocarcinoma, a staging laparoscopy is performed.
- Laparoscopy shows no evidence of peritoneal lesions or lymph node masses.

Progress of the patient

- This patient has no comorbidities that preclude major complex curative intent surgery.
- The oncologist decides on a course of pre-operative chemotherapy with cisplatin and 5-fluorouracil.

Most oesophageal surgeons in the UK would perform a staging laparoscopy for oesophageal carcinoma of the lower oesophagus if the histology is that of an adenocarcinoma, even if the cancer has not extended to the cardio-oesophageal junction.

SIGN guidelines recommend patients with operable oesophageal cancer who are treated by surgery to be considered for two cycles of pre-operative chemotherapy with cisplatin and 5-fluorouracil. There is evidence that neoadjuvant chemotherapy with cisplatin and 5-fluorouracil improves short-term survival over surgery alone. Other regimes are undergoing trial.

All patients should undergo careful pre-operative staging (Table 1) to identify those patients who are most likely to benefit from curative surgical treatment. The best long-term survival is associated with surgical therapy for oesophageal cancer without node involvement. However, reduction in the quality of life after surgery should be considered when discussing the treatment options, especially when pre-operative staging suggests that surgery is unlikely to be curative.

A careful assessment of fitness with emphasis on performance status and cardiorespiratory function should be conducted in all patients prior to surgery.

Clinical points

- Upper gastrointestinal endoscopy is the diagnostic procedure of choice for patients with dysphagia.
- A CT scan of the thorax, abdomen and pelvis is mandatory for pre-operative staging.
- All patients who are potential candidates for curative resection must have endoscopic ultrasound.
- A staging laparoscopy is considered for pre-operative staging in patients with oesophageal cancer with a possible gastric component.
- Positron emission tomography (PET) scans are increasingly being used in staging to look for occult metastases.
- Pre-operative chemotherapy with cisplatin and 5-fluorouracil is given to all patients prior to surgery if there are no contraindications for chemotherapy.

Most centres routinely perform blood gases, lung function tests, ECG/exercises, and an ECG +/- echocardiogram for pre-operative assessment.

It is recommended that all patients should undergo nutritional risk assessment pre-operatively by a dietician using a validated nutritional screening tool. Those considered as a high nutritional risk are given pre-operative nutritional support.

Pre-operative staging (Table 1)

This patient has an adenocarcinoma in the lower oesophagus. In general, adenocarcinomas commonly

Table 1. TNM staging of oesophageal carcinoma.

Category	Depth of infiltration	Node category	Regional lymph nodes
Tis	Carcinoma *in situ*.	NX	Nodes cannot be assessed.
T1	Invasion of lamina propria/submucosa.	N0	No node spread.
T2	Invasion of muscularis propria.	N1	Regional node metastases.
T3	Invasion of adventitia.	M0	No distant spread.
T4	Invasion of adjacent structures.	M1	Distant metastases.

occur in the distal one third of the oesophagus and squamous carcinomas occur in the proximal two thirds of the oesophagus.

The risk of developing an adenocarcinoma of the lower oesophagus is related to the duration and severity of gastro-oesophageal reflux and the progression of mucosal changes from Barrett's oesophagus to dysplasia and then to adenocarcinoma.

Early detection is the most important factor in determining the survival of patients with oesophageal cancer.

What is Barrett's oesophagus?

Barrett's oesophagus, which is also referred to as columnar-lined oesophagus (CLO) (BSG, 2005), is a condition which develops as a consequence of chronic gastro-oesophageal reflux. It is usually discovered during endoscopy performed to evaluate symptoms of gastro-oesophageal reflux disease.

As a consequence of longstanding reflux of the acidic gastric contents to the lower oesophagus, the lower oesophageal mucosa becomes 'adapted' to its new environment. This is done by changing its epithelial lining from an oesophageal type to a gastric type.

The stratified squamous epithelium which normally lines the distal oesophagus is replaced by an abnormal columnar epithelium that has intestinal features. This abnormal epithelium is referred to as intestinal metaplasia (IM). There is evidence of DNA damage in this mucosa which predisposes to malignancy.

Barrett's oesophagus affects mainly Caucasian men. It is considered to be a pre-cancerous lesion.

At endoscopy, Barrett's oesophagus is identified easily because of the change in colour between the normal oesophageal squamous-type epithelium and the columnar-type epithelium of Barrett's mucosa. Normal oesophageal mucosa has a pale glossy texture. The extension of the gastric type epithelium into the lower oesophagus appears a dull red (Figure 2).

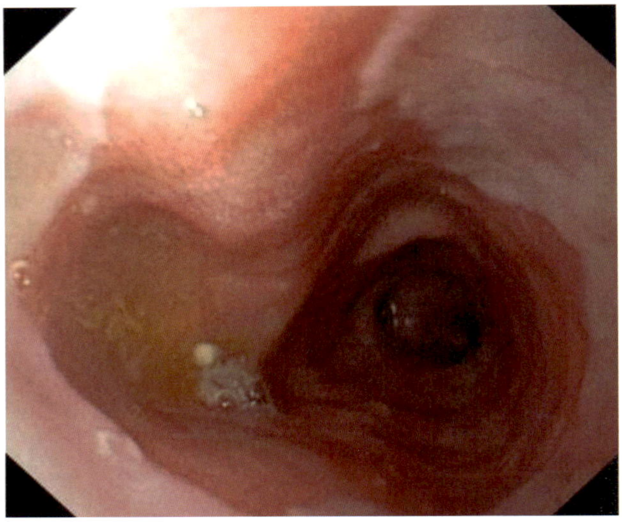

Figure 2. Endoscopic view of Barrett's oesophagus. ***Reproduced with permission from Hans Bjorknas, Gastrolab, Finland. www.gastrolab.net.***

Many changes have occurred since Norman Barrett described this condition in 1950.

Barrett's oesophagus was originally defined as the presence of gastric-type columnar epithelium which has extended circumferentially up to 3cm or more into the oesophagus which is visible macroscopically, when measured from the cardio-oesophageal junction.

Based on the present evidence, newer guidelines have carefully avoided the precise length and the need to have circumferential involvement.

The BSG guidelines (2005) define Barrett's oesophagus as any portion of the oesophagus which is replaced by metaplastic columnar epithelium which is visible macroscopically. In order to make a positive diagnosis of Barrett's oesophagus, a segment of columnar metapalsia of any length must be visible endoscopically above the oesophagogastric junction and confirmed histologically.

The American College of Gastroenterology guidelines insist on identifying the presence of IM. According to the latest UK guidelines this view is not supported by the UK pathological opinion.

What is the best strategy to prevent Barrett's oesophagus from progressing to oesophageal cancer?

There is no consensus as to the best strategy. The proposed strategies are:

- Anti-secretory drugs, in doses and combinations beyond which is required to treat the symptoms and signs of gastro-oesophageal reflux disease.
- Anti-reflux surgery.
- Endoscopic argon ablation of the metaplastic epithelium.
- Non-steroidal anti-inflammatory drugs that inhibit cyclo-oxygenase and its effects on cellular proliferation.
- Regular endoscopic surveillance.

Amongst the preventive strategies for cancer, only regular endoscopic surveillance has been recommended for routine clinical use by several guidelines and the colleges. Endoscopic surveillance has shown to reduce mortality from cancer in Barrett's oesophagus.

The strategy recommended by the American College of Gastroenterology is as follows:

- Patients with Barrett's oesophagus should have regular surveillance endoscopy. Gastro-oesophageal reflux disease should be treated before surveillance to minimise confusion caused by inflammation in the interpretation of dysplasia.
- Patients who have had two consecutive endoscopies that show no dysplasia should undergo surveillance by endoscopy every 3 years.
- If dysplasia is noted the finding should be verified by consultation with another expert pathologist.
- Patients with verified low-grade dysplasia after extensive biopsy sampling should have yearly surveillance endoscopy.
- In patients found to have high-grade dysplasia another endoscopy should be performed with extensive biopsy sampling (especially from areas with mucosal irregularity) to look for invasive cancer, and the histology slides should be interpreted by an expert pathologist. If there is verified, multifocal high-grade dysplasia, intervention (oesophagectomy) may be considered. This is because high-grade dysplasia is shown to be associated with a focus of invasive adenocarcinoma in 30-40% of patients.

Progress of the patient

- The respiratory function assessment shows no contraindication for major surgery.
- The echocardiogram demonstrates an ejection fraction of 70%.
- The FBC and liver, renal and coagulation profile are all normal.
- Pre-operative chest physiotherapy is applied.
- Four units of blood are cross-matched.
- Anti-thrombotic prophylaxis with low-molecular-weight heparin and peroperative calf compression is used.
- Antibiotic prophylaxis is given.
- The patient undergoes a two-stage (Ivor lewis) oesophagectomy 6 weeks after neoadjuvant treatment with cisplatin and 5-fluorouracil.

What surgical options are available for the treatment of oesophageal cancer?

- Two-stage oesophagectomy (Ivor Lewis operation).
- Three-stage oesophagectomy (McKeown operation).
- Transhiatal oesophagectomy (Orringer technique).
- Thoracoscopic-assisted oesophagectomy.

The main objective of surgery is to achieve an acceptable local clearance of the tumour which means an R0 resection (proximal, distal and circumferentinal margin clearance) and an adequate lymphadenectomy. This will also minimise the risk of a staging error. One important factor of the local spread of oesophageal cancer is its characteristic longitudinal submucosal spread. This pathological feature is seen in all types of oesophageal cancers. This accounts for a high rate of 'resection margin positivity' when resections are carried out without due consideration to the length of the oesophagus removed above and below the macroscopic margin of the tumour, because the tumour often extends submucosally beyond the macroscopic margin. Studies have supported the currently held view that the proximal resection margin of the tumour should ideally be 10cm above the macroscopic margin of the tumour and 5cm distal to it. Obviously, these ideal resection limits may need to be modified for more proximally located tumours.

A circumferential resection margin is shown as an independent risk factor for local recurrence following surgery. Local recurrence can be reduced in this situation by the use of postoperative radiotherapy and this should be strongly considered in squamous cell carcinoma, particularly when the proximal level of the tumour is high.

Adenocarcinoma of the lower oesophagus commonly infiltrates the gastric cardia, fundus and lesser curve. Some degree of gastric excision is essential in this situation.

Once the oesophagus and tumour are excised, continuity will be restored by bringing the stomach into the chest. When stomach is not available, colon interposition is the next most suitable conduit; jejunum is another option. Most surgeons favour a prevertebral route for reconstruction.

In an Ivor Lewis operation, a laparotomy is performed to mobilise the stomach, preserving its blood supply, and the oesophageal hiatus is widened. After closing the abdomen, the patient is re-positioned to the right lateral position and a posterolateral thoracotomy is performed. The tumour is mobilised with the regional lymph nodes, and the stomach is delivered into the chest through the widened oesophageal hiatus. An intrathoracic oesophago-gastric anastomosis is then performed.

The McKeown operation is a three-stage procedure where the mobilsed stomach is delivered up to the neck through the chest and the oesophago-gastric anastomosis is performed in the neck. Although it is technically a more demanding operation, the advantage claimed over the Ivor Lewis approach is that if an anastomotic leak occurs, it will occur in the neck outside the chest cavity.

In the transhiatal oesophagectomy, also called the Orringer technique, a thoracotomy is not performed. The oesophagus is approached through abdominal and neck incisions, the tumour and oesophagus are mobilised, the oesophagus is disconnected at the neck and delivered to the abdomen with the tumour. The gastric conduit is delivered through the prevertebral route to the neck and the oesophago-gastric anastomosis is performed in the neck.

The advantages of this technique are:

- A better postoperative recovery because of the absence of a chest incision.
- If a leak occurs at the anastomosis, it will occur in the neck, unlike in the Ivor Lewis approach where the leak occurs in the chest cavity.

However, transhiatal oesophagectomy is less popular as a cancer operation due to inadequate circumferential clearance and its lack of exposure to perform a lymphadenectomy. The dissection of the oesophagus and lymph nodes in the mediastinum in this operation is essentially a blind procedure using finger dissection through the neck incision and from the oesophageal hiatus.

The location of the tumour (upper, middle or lower) will determine the type of operative approach.

Laparoscopic and thoracoscopic-assisted oesophagectomies are being performed in specialised centres. With earlier detection, the newer minimally invasive techniques have found a place in the management of early lesions such as intramucosal cancers.

Superficial oesophageal cancer limited to the mucosa is treated with the endoscopic mucosal resection (EMR) technique if the patient is unfit for oesophagectomy.

Surgical treatment of resectable oesophageal cancers result in 5-year survival rates of 5-30%, with higher survival rates in patients with early-stage cancers.

High-volume centres performing oesophagectomies report 1-10% in-hospital mortality rates.

What options are available for the palliation of obstructing oesophageal cancer?

Endoscopically-placed metal oesophageal stents, laser treatment, photodynamic therapy and external beam radiotherapy are some of the palliative modalities available.

Oesophageal cancer has a poor prognosis. At the time of detection, many are not suitable for surgical resection. Palliative care constitutes an important aspect of the overall management of oesophageal cancer. The most distressing aspect of this condition is the fact that these patients do not lose appetite until later in the disease process but they cannot swallow.

What are the three main postoperative complications of oesophagectomy?

- Postoperative pulmonary complications.
- Anastomotic leak.
- Nutritional depletion.

Progress of the patient

- The immediate postoperative period is uneventful.
- Excellent pain control is achieved with a thoracic epidural line.
- Intensive chest physiotherapy and parenteral nutrition is commenced.
- A contrast study confirms an intact anastomosis on the fifth postoperative day and oral fluids and high protein enteral nutrition are started.
- The patient is discharged on the tenth postoperative day under the care of the specialist nurse practitioner and primary care physician, to be seen in the clinic in 4 weeks' time.

Suggested reading

1. Gillham CM, Reynolds BJ, Hollywood D. Predicting the response of localised oesophageal cancer to neoadjuvant chemoradiation. *World J Surg Oncol* 2007; 5: 7819-25.
2. Forshaw MJ, Gossage JA, Mason RC. Neoadjuvant chemotherapy for oesophageal cancer: the need for accurate response prediction and evaluation. *Surgeon* 2005; 1: 373-82.
3. Scottish Intercollegiate Guidelines Network. Management of oesophageal and gastric cancers. A national clinical guideline. SIGN, 2006.
4. British Society of Gastroenterology. Guidelines for diagnosis and management of Barrett's columnar-lined oesophagus. BSG, 2005.
5. Chandrasoma P. Controversies of the cardiac mucosa and Barrett's oesophagus. *Histopathology* 2005; 46: 361-73.
6. Sampliner RE and The Practice Parameters Committee of the American College of Gastroenterology. Updated guidelines for the diagnosis, surveillance, and therapy of Barrett's esophagus. *Am J Gastroenterol* 2002; 97: 1888-95

Self-assessment

Q1
EMQ

a. Upper GI endoscopy.
b. Upper GI endoscopy and endoscopic dilatation.
c. Contrast CT scan of the thorax, abdomen and pelvis.
d. Positron emission tomography (PET) scan.
e. Endoscopic ultrasound.

Select the most appropriate next step from the options given above for the case scenarios described below.

1. A 55-year-old ex-sailor presents with dysphagia of 4 weeks' duration.
2. A 60-year-old female with longstanding GORD presents with acute total dysphagia of 24-hour duration. A piece of chicken is found lodged at the lower end of the oesophagus above a benign-looking stricture.
3. At endoscopy a 45-year-old man is found to have a growth at 35cm which is biopsied.
4. A 75-year-old female with a lower one third oesophageal cancer has two small nodules in the right lung field on the CT scan.

Q2
SBA

A 60-year-old man underwent a curative intent transhiatal oesophagectomy for a squamous carcinoma of the lower oesophagus. An anastomotic leak occurred in the neck during the postoperative period but the fistula healed on conservative management. Four months after surgery he presents with dysphagia to solids.

What is the most likely clinical diagnosis?

a. Mediastinal lymphadenopathy.
b. Recurrence of cancer at the anastomosis.
c. Benign anastomotic stricture.
d. Carcinoma of the fundus of the stomach.
e. Abdominal adhesions.

Q3
True/False

Barrett's oesophagus:

a. Is associated with longstanding gastro-oesophageal reflux.
b. Is often asymptomatic.
c. Is lined by squamous epithelium.
d. Is pre-cancerous.
e. Precedes the development of squamous carcinoma of the oesophagus.

Q4
True/False

Risk factors for progression of Barrett's mucosa to adenocarcinoma include:

a. Smoking.
b. Obesity.
c. Early age of onset of GORD.
d. Duration of reflux.
e. Presence of mucosal damage (ulceration, stricture).

Answers overleaf

Self-assessment answers

Q1 1. (a), 2. (b), 3. (c), 4. (d).

Explanatory notes

d. A PET scan is a technique that is used for staging of oesophageal cancer and to detect recurrence after a primary tumour is removed.

The positron is the antimatter counterpart to the electron and, therefore, has the same mass as the electron but the opposite charge.

A PET scan is a functional scan, like a bone or thyroid scan, and uses the radioactive isotope fluorine-18 attached to a glucose molecule. The molecule is taken up by cells as glucose, so it localises in cells such as tumour cells that are metabolically active. The F-18 decays by emitting a positron.

PET imaging relies on the nature of the positron and positron decay.

A PET scan is very sensitive to the presence of tumour activity. A positive PET scan on the two lung nodules in this patient confirms metastatic disease.

Q2 (c).

Q3 a. (T), b. (T), c. (F), d. (T), e. (F).

Q4 a. (T), b. (T), c. (T), d. (T), e. (T).

Chapter 10

Occult gastrointestinal haemorrhage

Learning objectives

- To understand the assessment pathway of a patient with occult bleeding from the GI tract.
- To learn the investigative modalities available and to understand how such information is used in pre-operative staging.
- To learn the pre and postoperative tumour staging systems and the advantages of staging.
- To recollect the pathogenesis of colonic polyps and colon cancer.
- To appreciate the role of tumour markers in the diagnosis and postoperative surveillance of colon cancer.
- To appreciate the anatomical and pathological basis of surgery for right colon cancer.
- To learn the genetic basis of colorectal cancer.

Case scenario

A 75-year-old male presents with generalised tiredness and dyspnoea on mild exertion of 3 months' duration. He is on nitrates for ischaemic heart disease. During the last year he has been on laxatives intermittently for constipation but has not noticed a definite change in bowel habits. About 10 years ago, he underwent a polypectomy for a colonic polyp. He has no diabetes or hypertension.

On examination, he looks pale. His Hb is 9.5g/dL and his blood picture suggests a microcytic hypochromic anaemia. Two of the three faecal occult blood (FOB) samples are positive. The ECG shows no ischaemic changes and the chest X-ray is reported as normal.

The most likely clinical diagnosis: occult blood loss from the GI tract.

Occult GI bleeding may occur due to pathology in the upper GI system (oesophagus, stomach or duodenum) or from the lower GI tract. Occult blood loss can also be due to small intestinal pathology but this is less common than bleeding from the upper and lower GI tract. This patient has a history of colon polyps and positive occult blood. He has no history suggestive of any condition causing occult bleeding from the upper GI tract such as oesophageal varices, peptic ulceration or gastric cancer.

The lower GI tract is the most likely source of bleeding in patients who do not consume aspirin or non-steroidal anti-inflammatory drugs.

Anaemia is a common clinical presentation of right colon cancer in elderly patients.

The faecal occult blood (FOB) test detects blood in the stool that is not visible on gross inspection. Polyps and bowel cancers sometimes bleed. The FOB test works by detecting tiny amounts of blood which cannot normally be seen in bowel motions. The FOB test does not diagnose bowel cancer, but the results will indicate whether further investigation (usually a colonoscopy) is needed.

The current worldwide standard for FOB testing is the hemoccult slide test, a guaiac-based test (immunochemical), in which one side of a guaiac-impregnated paper is smeared with stool and tested by the addition of a few drops of developer solution (stabilised peroxide reagent) to the opposite side of the paper. The patient recovers stool from the toilet bowl using a wooden applicator, smears a small portion onto two windows of the card, and closes the cover. This is done on 3 successive days, and in the screening programmes, the cards are mailed for testing, as there is little degradation of reactive heme in the dry smeared specimens over a period of 1 week. Appearance of unequivocal blue colour of any intensity within 30 seconds is considered a positive test.

False-positive reactions are given by other materials that can catalyze the peroxidase reaction, including dietary peroxidases in vegetables and fruits, haemoglobin and myoglobin in red meats.

False-negative tests occur if high concentrations of reducing agents are present in the diet, especially ascorbic acid in citrus fruits and juices.

Drugs such as aspirin and non-steroidal anti-inflammatory agents, which often cause erosions and bleeding of gastric mucosa, also lead to positive tests. Therefore, the intake of meat, citrus fruits and juice should be eliminated for 3 days before and 3 days during the collection of stools.

Like all screening tests, the FOB test will not confirm or exclude colorectal cancer.

Faecal occult blood testing is the technique used by the National Health Service (NHS) bowel cancer screening programme in the UK. The NHS bowel cancer screening programme offers screening every 2 years to all men and women aged 60 to 69. The following is worthy of note:

- In general, around 98 in 100 people will receive a normal result. They will be invited for bowel cancer screening every 2 years if still within the eligible age range.
- About 2 in 100 people will receive an abnormal result. They will be offered a colonoscopy.
- About 5 in 10 people who have a colonoscopy will have a normal result.
- About 4 in 10 will be found to have a polyp, which if removed may prevent cancer developing.
- About 1 in 10 people will be found to have cancer when they have a colonoscopy.

Clinical points

- The NHS bowel cancer screening programme offers screening every 2 years to all men and women aged 60 to 69.
- To reduce false-positive and false-negative results, meat, citrus fruits and juices, aspirin and non-steroidal anti-inflammatory agents can be eliminated for 3 days before and 3 days during the collection of stools.
- Patients with abnormal results are offered colonoscopy.
- A negative FOB test does not exclude bowel cancer.

What is the next step?

- The patient undergoes a colonoscopy.

Colonoscopy is considered as the gold standard for the assessment of the colon. A video colonoscope is a 160cm long flexible tube which is inserted under sedation and opiate analgesia. The colonoscope may not reach the caecum in a small number of patients. The success of caecal intubation may be related to the experience of the endoscopist. In some patients technical issues such as sigmoid looping will also hamper the colonoscope reaching the caecum.

Complications associated with colonoscopy are perforation, bleeding and the risks of sedation including aspiration. Some elderly patients may be very sensitive to the combination of sedation and opiate analgesia.

Clinical points

- The lower GI tract is the most likely source of bleeding in patients who do not consume aspirin or non-steroidal anti-inflammatory drugs.
- Anaemia is a common clinical presentation of right colon cancer in the elderly.
- Patients should be informed of the risks and benefits of colonoscopy before consenting for the procedure.
- Colonoscopy is associated with a 1 in 1500 risk of perforation and a 1 in 150 risk of heavy bleeding.
- Colonoscopy carries a mortality of 1 in 10,000.

Progress of the patient

- Colonoscopy reveals a 1.5cm pedunculated polyp in the sigmoid colon. In the caecum, there is a 3.5cm ulcer with raised edges (Figure 1). The appearance is highly suggestive of a malignant ulcer. Multiple biopsies are obtained from the edges of the ulcer. The sigmoid polyp is removed by endoscopic polypectomy for histological analysis.

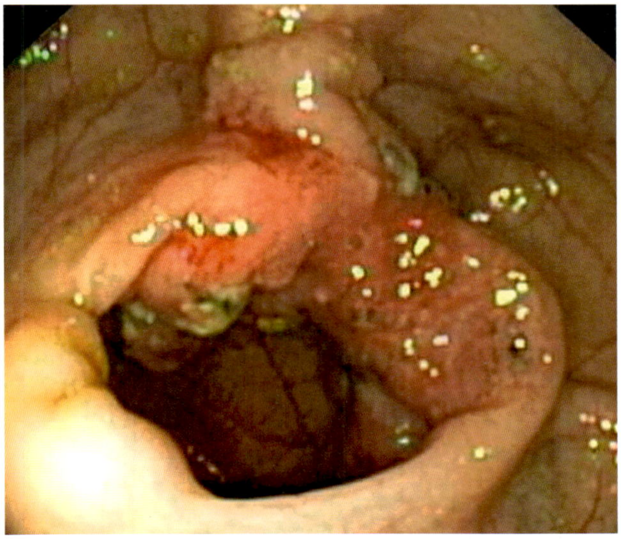

Figure 1. Cancer of the caecum. ***Reproduced with permission from Hans Bjorknas, Gastrolab, Finland. www.gastrolab.net.***

This patient has had polyps in the past. Therefore, it is likely that caecal cancer may have developed in the setting of a polyp. Most colorectal cancers develop on pre-existing polyps. As he had polyps in the past, he should have had regular colonoscopies to keep his colon under surveillance. The British Society of Gastroenterology (BSG) guidelines suggest that all patients with a history of polyps should be placed on a regular colonoscopic surveillance once in 5 years. However, the interval between surveillance colonoscopy will vary depending upon the perceived risk of malignant potential of the polyp and other factors such as a family history of colon cancer.

What are colon polyps?

Colon polyps are benign tumours that arise from the colonic epithelial cells. The two common types of polyps are hyperplastic polyps and adenomatous polyps. Hyperplastic polyps have no malignant potential, but adenomatous polyps are considered as pre-cancerous.

In general, the development of colon cancer from an adenomatous polyp follows a stepwise process. This process is referred to as the adenoma-carcinoma sequence. Colon cancer is one of the few cancers which has an identifiable pre-cancerous stage as a benign polyp. Complete excision of the polyp will reduce the cancer risk of the site of the polyp to zero.

Adenomas are classified either by their gross endoscopic appearance or on histology.

On endoscopic appearance they are classified as sessile which means flat and less mobile or pedunculated which means that the polyp has a stalk. Sessile polyps commonly have a delicate villous surface much like the surface of a sea anemone. Pedunculated polyps have a lobulated head with a red/brown surface. This is how they appear on colonoscopy.

Histologically, adenomatous polyps are classified into three types: villous, tubulovillous or tubular (Figures 2 and 3) .

It is not possible to predict the presence of a carcinoma on the gross appearance of a polyp. In general, the malignant potential of a polyp depends on three factors:

- Size of the polyp. The larger (more than 1cm) the polyp, the higher the malignant potential.
- Type of the polyp. Villous adenomas have the highest malignant potential.
- Degree of epithelial dysplasia. Severely dysplastic polyps have a high malignant potential.

By definition, all adenomas are composed of dysplastic epithelium. The pathologist will report on the degree of dysplasia as mild, moderate or severe.

Progress of the patient

- Whilst the biopsy is awaited, the patient has a contrast CT scan of the thorax, abdomen and pelvis.
- Blood is sent off to test for carcino-embryonic antigen (CEA).
- The contrast CT shows a caecal tumour which appears to be confined to the caecal wall (Figure 4). Two enlarged lymph nodes are seen in the mesocolon. There is no evidence of liver, peritoneal or pulmonary metastases.
- The CEA level is <2µg/L (normal up to 2.5µg/L).

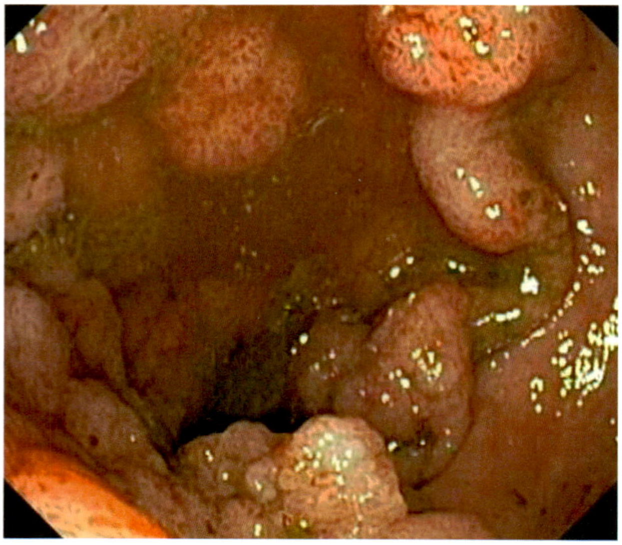

Figure 2. Villous adenomata of the rectum. *Reproduced with permission from Hans Bjorknas, Gastrolab, Finland. www.gastrolab.net.*

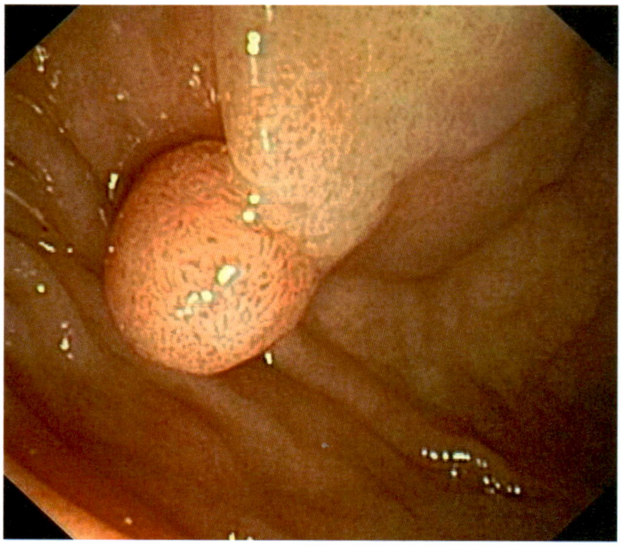

Figure 3. Tubular adenoma of the sigmoid colon. *Reproduced with permission from Hans Bjorknas, Gastrolab, Finland. www.gastrolab.net.*

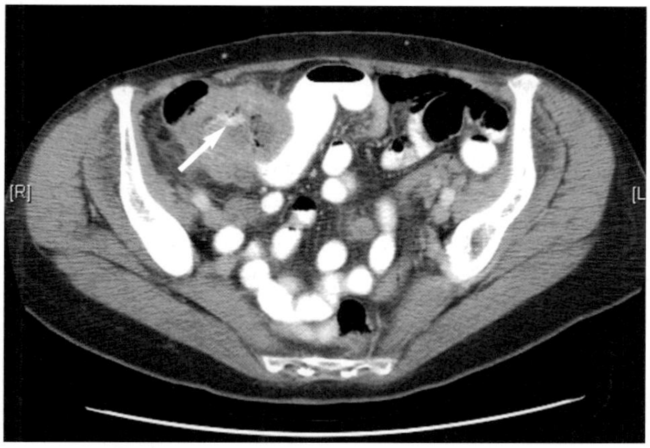

Figure 4. CT scan showing a caecal cancer (arrow). ***Reproduced with permission from Dr M Tee, Consultant Radiologist, Leighton Hospital, Crewe, UK.***

Progress of the patient

- Histology of the polyp removed from the sigmoid colon is reported as a tubular adenoma with moderate dysplasia. The excision appears to be complete. The caecal growth is reported as a moderately differentiated adenocarcinoma.
- The patient is discussed at the colorectal MDT meeting.
- He undergoes a right hemicolectomy.

This patient has already had a colonoscopy and the cancer in the caecum is confirmed histologically. Therefore, is there a need for a contrast CT scan of the thorax, abdomen and pelvis?

It is good practice to stage colon cancers prior to definitive treatment. A CT scan is done for this purpose.

Colon cancers commence in the mucosa and from this point of origin, will spread locally in three directions. It spreads longitudinally along the bowel, circumferentially around the bowel wall like a constriction ring and radially across the bowel wall into the surrounding structures.

In the colon there are no lymphatic channels in the epithelium, lamina propria or muscularis mucosa. The main lymphatic channels are in the submucosa. Therefore, a tumour breaking through the muscularis mucosa to the submucosa is an important finding as it is in the submucosa that lymph channels are found in abundance. The cells entering this maze of lymphatic channels have the potential to spread further, to the regional mesenteric lymph nodes and to distant sites such as the liver and lung once it reaches this plane. The local infiltration will continue to involve the muscularis propria, adjacent organs, peritoneum and abdominal wall.

At colonoscopy, the surgeon will visualise the cancer and establish accurate information on the length of the lesion including the extent of longitudinal and circumferential spread. The extent of radial spread cannot be obtained at colonoscopy; a CT scan is useful to gain this information.

There is a risk of bowel obstruction with extensive circumferential involvement. A contrast CT scan will be highly valuable to assess the degree of bowel obstruction. It is also useful to detect if there is any further spread to the regional lymph nodes and to distant sites.

If this information is available, better decisions can be made. For example, if the bulk of the tumour is large, or if the tumour is shown to invade the adjacent organs or abdominal wall, the oncologist might suggest a neoadjuvant protocol to downsize the tumour prior to surgical intervention.

If the contrast CT indicates significant bowel obstruction, the patient will need urgent surgical intervention to prevent perforation of the bowel. Perforation of the bowel carries a high mortality.

Detection of widespread metastases at initial detection will have a significant bearing on the management approach.

What is the role of a double-contrast barium enema in the management of such a patient?

A double-contrast barium enema is a commonly used modality to assess the colon in many countries

(Figure 5). With the advent of colonoscopy, CT colography and the contrast CT scan, however, the use of barium enemas has declined in specialised centres.

When colonoscopic assessment of the right colon is not possible due to technical reasons, a double-contrast barium study can be a valuable tool. However, in a patient with a previous history of colon polyps presenting with symptoms of anaemia, a colonoscopy is the next logical step because small polyps can be missed on barium studies. Also, during colonoscopy biopsies can be obtained to assist a definitive diagnosis and the polyps can be removed.

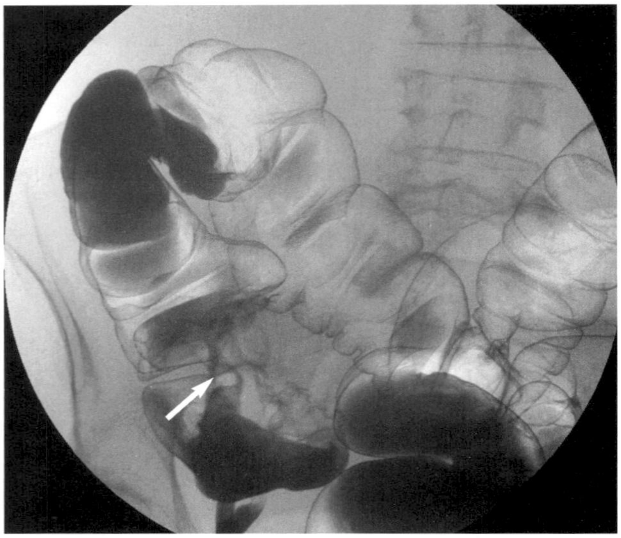

Figure 5. Barium enema showing a caecal cancer (arrow). ***Reproduced with permission from Dr M Tee, Consultant Radiologist, Leighton Hospital, Crewe, UK.***

What is carcino-embryonic antigen (CEA)?

Carcino-embryonic antigen is a glycoprotein which is produced during the development of the fetus. The production of CEA stops before birth and is found only in very small quantities in the blood of healthy adults. Cancer of the colon usually secretes CEA and therefore it can be used as a tumour marker.

Is CEA helpful in the diagnosis of colorectal cancer?

CEA cannot be used independently to establish a diagnosis of colorectal cancer.

Is CEA helpful in monitoring the cancer treatment?

The regular assay of plasma CEA is the best non-invasive technique for postoperative surveillance of patients to detect the recurrence of colorectal cancer.

Following complete surgical removal of cancer, the elevated plasma CEA value will usually return to normal by 6 weeks. The failure to observe a reduction of a previously elevated pre-operative CEA is strongly indicative of the presence of a residual tumour.

CEA becomes significantly elevated before metastatic disease can be detected by clinical or other diagnostic measures.

Is CEA useful as a screening tool for colorectal cancer?

CEA is not recommended for screening of colorectal cancer.

Clinical points

- Following complete surgical excision of the cancer, an elevated CEA will usually return to normal by 6 weeks.
- The regular assay of plasma CEA is the best non-invasive technique for postoperative surveillance of patients to detect the recurrence of colorectal cancer.
- CEA levels often become significantly elevated before metastatic disease can be detected by clinical or radiological methods.
- CEA is not recommended for colon cancer screening.

What is a right hemicolectomy?

The principal objective of surgery for colon cancer is to remove the tumour completely with its blood supply and lymphatic drainage. Blood supply to the caecum is from the ileocolic artery and right colic artery. The venous and lymphatic drainage follow the same pathway. At the hepatic flexure, the arterial arcades of the right colic artery anastomose with the branches of the middle colic artery. As shown in Figure 6, the extent of bowel removed in a right hemicolectomy operation involves 2-3cm of the distal ileum, the ileocaecal valve, the caecum, the ascending colon, the hepatic flexure and the right one third of the transverse colon with a segment of mesocolon containing the territorial blood vessels, lymph channels and lymph nodes. A V-shaped segment of the mesocolon is excised in continuity with the previously described segment of bowel with the apex of the V at the origin of the ileocolic and middle colic artery. The duodenum and right ureter are identified to prevent accidental injury. Mobilisation of the hepatic flexure can be difficult in some patients.

The pathologist will take sections from the main specimen to accurately stage the disease and assess to what extent the bowel wall is involved. They will report on the completeness of the excision by assessing the presence or absence of cancer cells in three main sites of the resected specimen of the colon or rectum. These are:

- Proximal resection margin of the tumour.
- Distal resection margin of the tumour.
- Circumferential resection margin.

For proximal and distal margin clearance, a 5cm margin from the macroscopic edge of the tumour is considered ideal. However, recent literature suggests that a macroscopic clearance of 1cm is acceptable for low rectal cancers.

The phrase 'circumferential resection margin' is used to indicate the lateral clearance of the tumour which is the extent of the radial spread.

Two factors which are shown to be associated with an increased risk of local recurrence of tumour after surgery are:

- Involvement of the circumferential resection margin by the tumour.

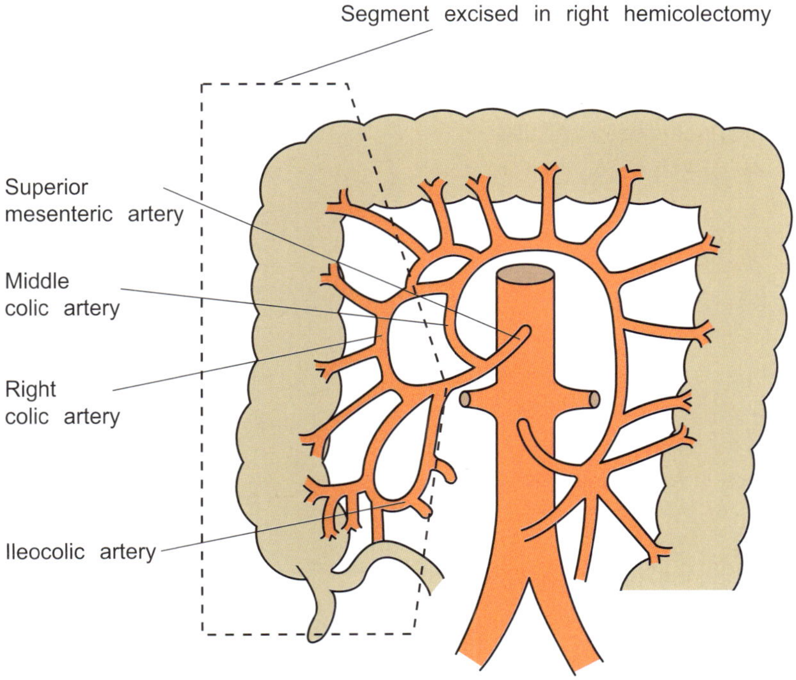

Figure 6. Surgical anatomy of the right colon for right hemicolectomy.

- Lympho-vascular involvement (presence of tumour cells in the blood vessels or lymphatics).

The pathologist will also carefully dissect all the lymph nodes in the specimen to assess the nodal involvement. They will report on the total number of lymph nodes 'harvested' from the specimen and indicate how many of them contain cancer cells.

According to good practice guidelines (The Royal College of Pathologists, 2007), a histopathological report should contain a minimum of 12 lymph nodes.

The lymph nodes in the mesocolon are commonly described in three groups. The epicolic lymph nodes are the nodes which are located adjacent to the large bowel wall. These nodes are hidden in the appendix epiploicae, the fat lobules on the bowel wall. Another group of nodes, known as paracolic nodes, lie along the mesenteric side of the colon. Therefore, bowel cancers which are located on the mesenteric border are closer to the lymph node stations, as well as to the larger blood and lymphatic vessels. The nodes which are found around the origin of the main vessel of the draining territory are referred to as the apical nodes.

Progress of the patient

- The postoperative period is uneventful.
- Histology of the resected specimen is reported as a well differentiated adenocarcinoma. All three excision margins are clear (PT3, Dukes' B).

What is Dukes' classification?

The Dukes' classification deals with the invasion of the tumour through the bowel wall. Therefore, the entire specimen of the resected bowel is required for this purpose. It is regarded as a valuable prognostic indicator.

The original Dukes' classification placed patients into one of three categories as Stage A, B, and C:

- A. The tumour is confined to the bowel wall.
- B. The tumour infiltrates through the bowel wall.
- C. The tumour has spread to the lymph nodes.

This system was subsequently modified by Astler-Coller. A fourth stage called Stage D was included to indicate distant metastases.

More recently, the International Union against Cancer (UICC) and the American Joint Committee on Cancer (AJCC) introduced the TNM staging system (Table 1). The TNM system is considered as a more accurate classification because it takes into account the details of the local extension.

Table 1. TNM staging system (tumour, node, metastases)

Tumour

- Tis (carcinoma *in situ*): the tumour is confined to the mucosa; also referred to as intra-mucosal carcinoma.
- T1: the tumour has invaded the submucosa.
- T2: the tumour has invaded the muscularis propria. This is the main muscle layer which is also referred to as muscularis externa.
- T3: the tumour has penetrated through the muscularis propria into the subserosa or pericolic fat but not into the peritoneal cavity or other organs.
- T4: the tumour has directly invaded through the muscle wall into the visceral peritoneum or has invaded other adjacent organs.

Lymph nodes

- N0: no regional lymph node metastases.
- N1: metastases in 1 to 3 regional lymph nodes.
- N2: metastases in 4 or more regional lymph nodes.

Metastases

- M0: no distant metastases.
- M1: distant metastases present.

Table 2. A comparison between TNM and Dukes' classification.

AJCC/TNM	DUKES
◆ Tis. Intra-mucosal carcinoma or carcinoma *in situ.*	◆ This is not regarded as a cancer.
◆ T1. The tumour has invaded the submucosa.	◆ A
◆ T2. The tumour has invaded muscle, N0, M0.	◆ A
◆ T3. The tumour has traversed through the muscle and broken through the outer covering.	◆ B
◆ T4. The tumour has broken though the outer covering into adjacent tissue or organs but there is no lymph node involvement or distant metastases.	◆ B
◆ T1 N1 M0 or T2 N1 M0 or T3 N1 M0.	◆ C
◆ T4 N1 M0 or any with N2. (N1= 1-3 nodes) (N2= 4 or more nodes). (In other words any T, any N, M0).	◆ C
◆ Any T, any N but with M the tumour has spread to distant sites such as the liver or lung.	◆ C

A comparison between TNM and Dukes' classification is shown in Table 2 and Figure 7. At a MDT meeting the pathologist may present a case as pT3 N1 as the primary tumour has locally extended through the muscularis propria to involve the serosa. As the lymph node is involved this makes it a Dukes' C carcinoma. The TNM classification gives more accurate details.

Clinical points

- The established basis for colorectal cancer staging at present is the TNM system.
- The TNM system takes into account the depth of tumour invasion through the bowel wall, the extent of lymph node involvement and the presence of distant metastases.

Clinical points

- With present investigative modalities such as CT, MRI and EUS, the precise extent of bowel wall involvement and distant spread can be assessed pre-operatively.
- Dukes' staging is still used sporadically.

Is there a benefit from adjuvant chemotherapy?

Although the benefit from adjuvant chemotherapy has been clearly established in patients with Dukes' C colon cancer, such benefit has been questioned in patients with Dukes' B disease with regards to the

Tis Because Tis is not a carcinoma, the Dukes' comparison cannot be given

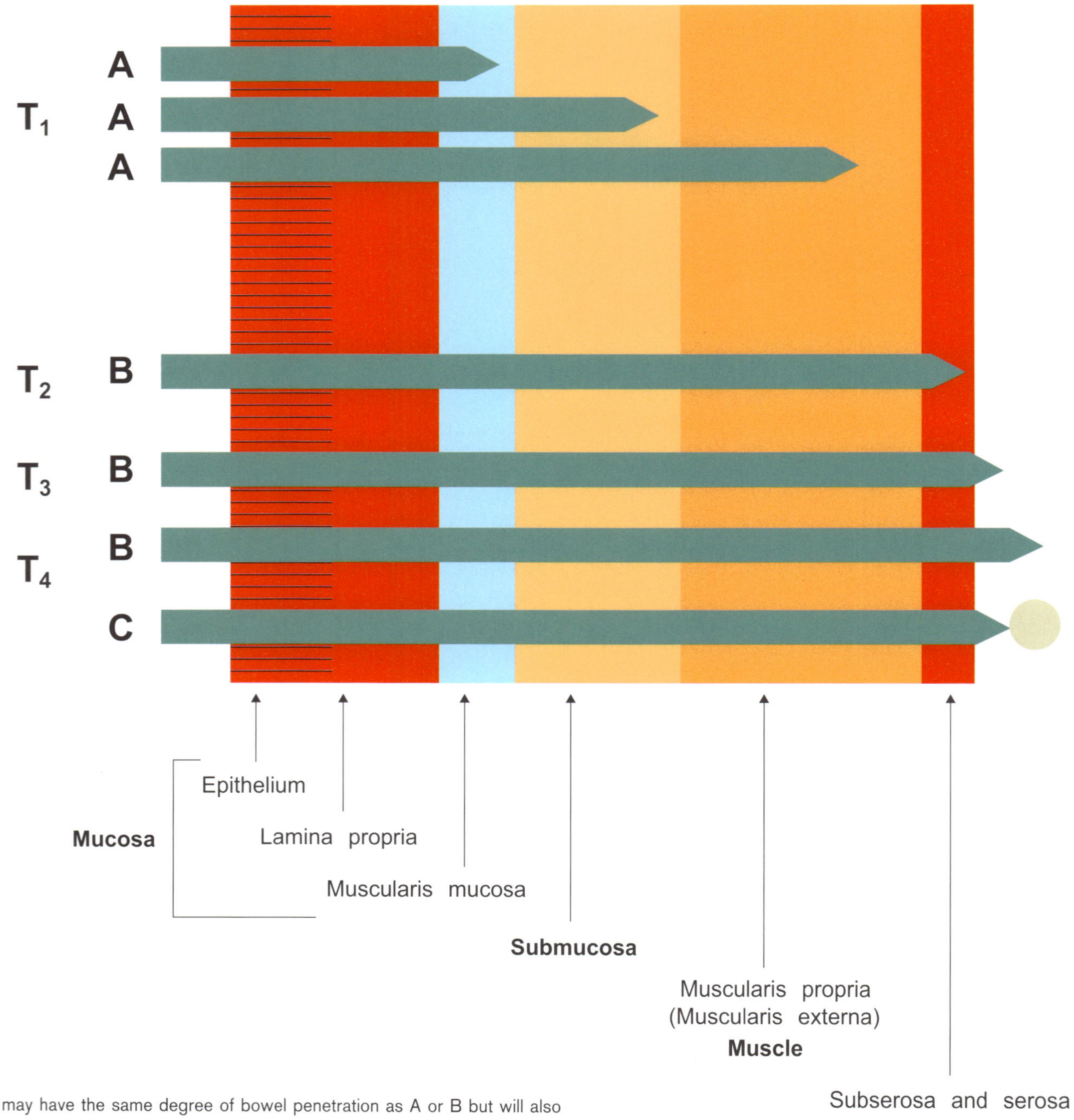

C may have the same degree of bowel penetration as A or B but will also have lymph node involvement. It is important to appreciate that the word 'mucosa' refers to 3 layers: the epithelium, lamina propria and muscularis mucosa

Figure 7. A comparison between TNM and Dukes' classification.

overall disease-free and recurrence-free survival improvement. However, some oncologists use chemotherapy for Dukes' B colon cancer regardless of the presence or absence of other clinical prognostic factors.

Progress of the patient

- The final histology is discussed at the MDT meeting. He is seen in the oncology clinic 2 weeks after surgery. Considering the age and histological grading the oncologist decides not to treat him with chemotherapy.

Suggested reading

1. Scottish Intercollegiate Guidelines Network. Management of colorectal cancer - a national clinical guideline. SIGN, 2003: 67.
2. UK bowel cancer incidence statistics. Cancer Research, UK, 2005.
3. Hewitson P, Glasziou P, Irwig L, Towler B, Watson E. Screening for colorectal cancer using the faecal occult blood test: an update. *Cochrane Database of Systematic Reviews* 2006; 4: CD001216.
4. Williams GT Quirke P, Shepherd NA. Standards and data sets for reporting cancers. Data set for colorectal cancer, 2nd edition. The Royal College of Pathologists, 2007.
5. Vasen HF, Watson P, Mecklin JP, Lynch HT. The Netherlands Foundation for the Detection of Hereditary Tumours, Leiden, The Netherlands. New clinical criteria for hereditary nonpolyposis colorectal cancer (HNPCC, Lynch syndrome) proposed by the International Collaborative Group on HNPCC. *Gastroenterology* 1999; 116(6): 1453-6.

Self-assessment

Q1
EMQ

With regard to colon polyps:

a. Hyperplastic polyp.
b. Adenomatous polyp.
c. Villous adenoma.
d. Pseudopolyp.

Select the most appropriate characteristic from below to match the type of colon polyp given above.

1. Dysplastic epithelium.
2. Associated with ulcerative colitis.
3. High malignant potential.
4. No malignant potential.

Q2
SBA

An elderly male presents with generalised tiredness and dyspnoea on exertion of 3 months' duration. He has no history of dyspepsia, bleeding per rectum, long-term use of non-steroidal anti-inflammatory agents or ischaemic heart disease.

On examination, he looks pale. His Hb is 7.5g/dL. The blood picture suggests microcytic hypochromic anaemia and the renal profile is normal. Two of the three occult blood samples are positive. The ECG shows no ischaemic changes. A chest X-ray is reported as normal.

What is the most likely site of occult blood loss?

a. Lower oesophagus.
b. Stomach.
c. Duodenum.
d. Small bowel.
e. Colon.

Q3
SBA

What is the most useful investigation to arrive at a definitive diagnosis as to the cause of his occult blood loss?

a. Contrast CT scan of the abdomen and pelvis.
b. Upper GI endoscopy.
c. Colonoscopy.
d. Barium enema.
e. Ultrasound scan.

Q4
SBA

Which of the following conditions has the highest risk of developing colorectal cancer?

a. Adenomatous polyposis coli (APC).
b. Family history of colon cancer.
c. History of ulcerative colitis.
d. History of colonic Crohn's disease.
e. History of solitary rectal adenoma.

Q5
True/False

Colonoscopy:

a. Is commonly performed under sedation.
b. Carries a 1 in 1500 risk of bowel perforation.
c. Needs antibiotic prophylaxis prior to the procedure.
d. Has no therapeutic potential.
e. Is expected to visualise the caecum and intubation of the caecum is best confirmed by a positive ileal biopsy.

Q6
True/False

Carcino-embryonic antigen:

a. Is not present in the blood of healthy adults.
b. Is used as an independent marker to establish a diagnosis of colon cancer.
c. Is the best non-invasive investigation for postoperative surveillance of patients to detect recurrence of colorectal cancer.
d. Becomes significantly elevated before metastatic disease can be detected by clinical or radiological methods.
e. Is recommended as a screening investigation for colorectal cancer.

Q7
True/False

Colonoscopy is useful to assess:

a. The extent of the longitudinal spread of colon cancer.
b. Circumferential spread of colon cancer.
c. Radial spread of colon cancer.
d. Nodal involvement of colon cancer.
e. Site of colon cancer.

Answers overleaf

Self-assessment answers

Q1 1. (b), 2. (d), 3. (c), 4. (a).

Explanatory notes

By definition, all adenomatous polyps consist of dysplastic epithelium. The degree of dysplasia may be mild to severe.

Areas of mucosal ulceration in ulcerative colitis heal by granulation tissue. The raised areas of inflammatory tissue during the attempted healing process resemble polyps. These are called pseudopolyps. Pseudopolyps are merely inflammatory tissue and have no malignant potential. But ulcerative colitis is a pre-malignant condition.

Of the adenomatous polyps, villous adenomas have the highest malignant potential.

Hyperplastic polyps have no malignant potential.

Q2 (e).

Q3 (c).

Q4 (a).

Explanatory notes

a. Adenomatous polyposis coli (APC) is associated with almost 100% risk of developing colorectal cancer in later life. The APC gene is situated in chromosome 5. APC has an autosomal dominant inheritance and is characterised by the presence of hundreds of polyps in the colon. A total colectomy is indicated in these patients after the second or third decade. However, APC constitutes about 1% of all colorectal cancers.

b. Individuals with a family history of colorectal cancer have an increased risk of developing the disease. The risk is greater with early age of onset and with multiple affected relatives.

Most patients with a strong family history of colorectal cancer belong to a group with the condition called hereditary non-polyposis colorectal cancer (HNPCC).

HNPCC is a hereditary syndrome. It is caused when a person inherits a mutation in one of six mismatch repair genes. Individuals with HNPCC have a much higher risk of developing colon cancer than the general population.

The term HNPCC may be a misnomer for students. The word 'non-polyposis' may give an erroneous impression that these patients develop colon cancers without the polyp stage. HNPCC patients also develop colon polyps and polyps; the cancer sequence is recognised in HNPCC. The word 'non-polyposis' is used to differentiate HNPCC from adenomatous polyposis coli (APC).

The second reason for the confusion is because of the term 'colorectal cancer'. HNPCC mutations predispose not only to colorectal cancer but also to cancers at least in seven other areas including the endometrium, stomach, ovaries, small bowel, hepatobiliary and uroepithelial area, and the brain.

HNPCC is also known as Lynch syndrome. The term HNPCC was introduced to accurately characterise patients who were formally described as having Lynch syndrome. HNPCC is subdivided into Lynch syndrome I and II. Lynch syndrome I is also referred to as family colon cancer and Lynch syndrome II is associated with other cancers of the GI tract and in other organs.

HNPCC is responsible for approximately 5% of all colorectal cancers. Most HNPCC tumours occur in young patients. They are mostly found in the right colon.

HNPCC is due to inherited mutations in the mismatch repair genes, which degrade the self-repair capability of DNA or the mismatch repair mechanism. The mismatch repair genes identified are MLH1, MSH2, MSH6, MSH3, PMS1 and PMS2. The penetrance for these genes for colorectal cancer is approximately 80% and is less for other cancers.

Inherited defects in these genes results in micro-satellite instability.

What is meant by the self-repair capability of DNA?

The replication of DNA is a continuous process in the human body when cells continue to multiply. The nucleus of a cell contains DNA strands with millions of base pairs. When DNA replicates, mistakes do occur when the base pairs mismatch. It is like a typist typing millions of different sequences all the time. Obviously mistakes are bound to happen with repetition. But the proteins produced by the DNA repair genes will scan all newly formed DNA strands before the final print to identify the segments or base pairs that are defective and are promptly repaired. If the repair genes are defective (mismatch repair genes), the process will fail which results in the accumulation of defective DNA strands.

Genes are segments of DNA responsible for a production of a protein. However, there are segments of DNA in a long DNA strand that have no specific function. These areas are called micro-satellite regions. Micro-satellite instability is seen when the DNA mismatch repair genes are defective.

Pathologically it is easy to detect micro-satellite instability in a tumour specimen than trying to isolate the defective genes.

The revised Amsterdam criteria (Amsterdam II), identifies families likely to have HNPCC.

These criteria are:

- At least three relatives should have developed HNPCC-associated cancers such as colorectal cancer, endometrial cancer or cancers of the small intestine, ureter or renal pelvis.
- One patient should be a first degree relative of the other two.
- At least two successive generations should be affected.
- At least one tumour should be diagnosed at less than 50 years of age.

Some believe that the Amsterdam criteria are too stringent.

Q5 a. (T), b. (T), c. (F), d. (F), e. (T).

Q6 a. (F), b. (F), c. (T), d. (T), e. (F).

Q7 a. (T), b. (T), c. (F), d. (F), e. (T).

Chapter 11

Altered bowel habits

Learning objectives

- To learn the diagnostic work-up of a patient with altered bowel habits.
- To learn the value and limitations of CT, MRI and EUS in the diagnosis of rectal cancer.
- To learn the pre-operative staging of colorectal cancer.
- To learn the anatomical and pathological basis of total mesorectal excision (TME) and its value.
- To appreciate the role of radiotherapy in the management of rectal cancer.

Case scenario

An 80-year-old lady presents with a history of increased frequency of stools of 2 months' duration. She has about 4-6 motions a day. She also has a frequent desire to defecate but often produces little loose stools, sometimes mixed with mucus and blood. She has no anal pain but experiences lower abdominal colic when she feels the urge to pass a stool. During this period, she has lost a stone in weight and is scared to eat because of the abdominal colic.

She has Type 1 diabetes and hypertension. She has had a myocardial infarction 15 years ago. She is on antihypertensive medication, oral hypoglycaemics and aspirin.

On examination she appears thin, frail and has a mild pallor. The abdominal examination is unremarkable. An ulcerated mass is felt by the finger on digital rectal examination and blood-stained mucus is observed on the examination finger.

The most likely clinical diagnosis: rectal cancer.

The recent alteration of bowel habits, with an increased frequency of loose stools, a frequent urge for defecation and the presence of blood and mucus in stools, all point to a sinister pathology in the rectum. The presence of blood at the tip of the examination finger indicates that the most likely source of blood is the ulcerative lesion felt in the lower rectum.

Haemorrhoids commonly present with fresh rectal bleeding and this clinical picture is very unlikely to be due to haemorrhoids.

Colicky abdominal pain prior to defecation suggests a possible obstruction low down in the colon or in the upper rectum. This clinical picture is frequently seen in patients with partially occluding cancers at the rectosigmoid junction or in the upper rectum.

The guidelines for urgent referral from primary care for patients suspected of having a bowel tumour are:

- Rectal bleeding without anal symptoms in patients over 60 for more than 6 weeks.
- Loose or more frequent stools in patients over 60 for more than 6 weeks.
- Loose or more frequent stools and rectal bleeding at any age.
- A palpable rectal mass.
- A palpable abdominal mass.
- Iron-deficient anaemia.

These are important signs and symptoms but these symptoms should never be accepted as an adequate history. A more comprehensive system of questions has been shown to give greater accuracy. One way of doing this is to use a Patient Consultation Questionnaire (PCQ) asking multiple facets of individual symptoms and this can be completed by the patient prior to seeing the clinician. From this a score (Selva Score) can be derived by weighting the symptoms and symptom complexes in relation to cancer outcome. This, in conjunction with the clinical findings, can guide the prioritisation of the patient and the pathways of investigation.

Progress of the patient

- A rigid sigmoidoscopy is performed. An ulcerative growth is seen at 7cm from the anal verge. Several biopsies are obtained for histology.
- Blood is collected for an FBC, a liver, renal and coagulation profile, blood group and for CEA levels.
- A date for colonoscopy, a CT scan of the thorax, abdomen and pelvis, and a pelvic MRI scan are arranged for pre-operative staging of the tumour.
- The patient and her husband are informed that the symptoms are very likely to be due to a lesion in the rectum which needs further assessment. She is advised about bowel preparation prior to colonoscopy. She is also introduced to the specialist colorectal nurse.

What is rigid sigmoidoscopy?

A rigid sigmoidoscope is a metal or plastic tube which is 25cm in length with a light source to visualise the rectum. With the patient in the left lateral position the scope is inserted into the anal canal and guided to the rectum. Air is injected to distend the rectum. Although it is called a sigmoidoscope, it is uncommon to be able to gain entry to the sigmoid colon passing the rectosigmoid junction, as the injected air distends and elongates the rectum.

If a full colonoscopy is arranged, what is the need for this procedure?

This patient has symptoms and signs suggestive of a rectal cancer and, if found, this needs histological confirmation. The processing and reporting of biopsies will take about a week. Rectal lesions can be visualised with the rigid sigmoidoscope and biopsies can be obtained to speed up the process. During this period, colonoscopy, a CT scan of the thorax, abdomen and pelvis, and an MRI scan of the pelvis can be performed to obtain further information to confirm the diagnosis and to stage the disease.

Many 'one-stop' colorectal clinics have facilities for rigid or flexible sigmoidoscopy.

What is bowel preparation?

As colonoscopy involves the passage of a scope up to the caecum, a clean bowel is necessary to obtain a clear view. Most of the agents used to clean the colon are strong laxatives which act locally with little or no systemic absorption. Two of the commonly used agents are polyethylene glycol and sodium picosulphate. One sachet of polyethylene glycol is dissolved in one litre of water and the patient is requested to drink the litre of fluid in about an hour. One sachet of sodium picosulphate is dissolved in a glass of water. The patient is instructed to commence bowel preparation on the previous evening if the colonoscopy is planned for the morning. Two or three sachets may be required.

What is an MRI scan? Why is there a need to obtain both a CT scan of the thorax, abdomen and pelvis, and an MRI of the pelvis in this patient?

Magnetic resonance imaging is a special scan which uses the magnetic properties of human tissue. Therefore, unlike X-rays or CT scans, there is no radiation hazard involved with MRI.

The human body is filled with biological magnets. The most responsive is the hydrogen atom. The body is placed in a strong magnetic field and the hydrogen atoms are stimulated by radiofrequency energy. Radiofrequency stimulation is then terminated and the movement of hydrogen atoms are listened to, at a special resonant frequency. The transmitted signal is detected and serves as the basis to create internal images of the body using computer principles.

MRI is better than a CT scan to show soft tissue details. MRI will also demonstrate how deeply the tumour has grown into the body tissues locally. MRI provides a better picture than a CT scan in the pelvis and is, therefore, a better tool than CT to assess the local spread of rectal cancer. Contrast is injected before an MRI scan in order to obtain clearer pictures.

MRI cannot be performed if the patient has metals in the body, e.g. hip replacement.

Transrectal endoscopic ultrasound (EUS) is also an excellent alternative modality to investigate the local extension of rectal cancers.

Clinical points

- MRI provides details of the local spread of the rectal cancer and is a better tool than CT for this purpose.
- Unlike CT, there is no radiation hazard with MRI scans.
- Transrectal endoscopic ultrasound is also an excellent tool to assess local extension of the rectal cancer.
- Thoracic and abdominal CT scans will provide information of the spread of the tumour to distant sites such as the liver and lung.

Progress of the patient

- Histology confirms a moderately differentiated adenocarcinoma. Colonoscopy shows an ulcerated rectal growth involving 50% of the circumference, with the lower margin at 3cm from the dentate line. The length of the tumour is 3.5cm.
- The colonoscope is negotiated through the tumour (Figure 1). A clear view is obtained up to the caecum. No polyps or synchronous tumours are identified.

Progress of the patient

- MRI shows a T3 tumour (extending into the muscularis propria). Two enlarged mesorectal nodes are seen but do not have the radiological characteristics of malignant nodes.
- A CT scan of the thorax, abdomen and pelvis confirms the rectal cancer.
- There is no evidence of intraperitoneal disease or distant spread.

What is the next step?

- The patient is discussed at the MDT meeting.
- The MRI is reported as a T3 tumour (Figure 2).
- A course of pre-operative radiotherapy to downstage the tumour and an abdominoperineal resection (APR) is proposed as the definitive plan.
- The unit policy is to perform a 'specimen-based' dissection to achieve a total mesorectal excision.

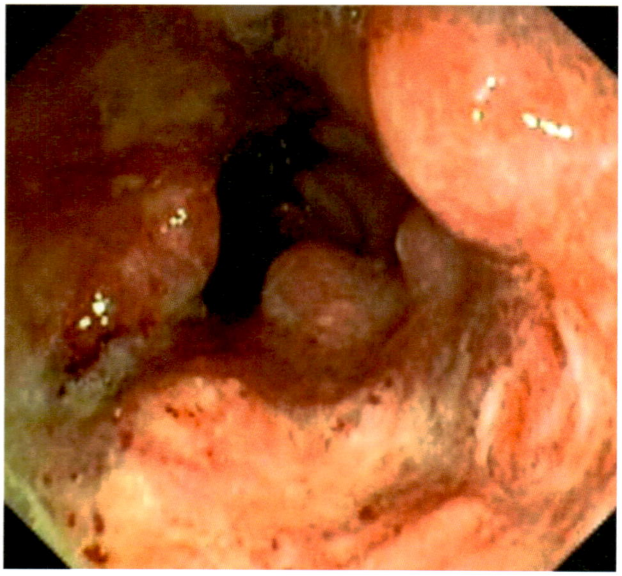

Figure 1. Endoscopic view of a rectal cancer. *Reproduced with permission from Hans Bjorknas, Gastrolab, Finland. www.gastrolab.net.*

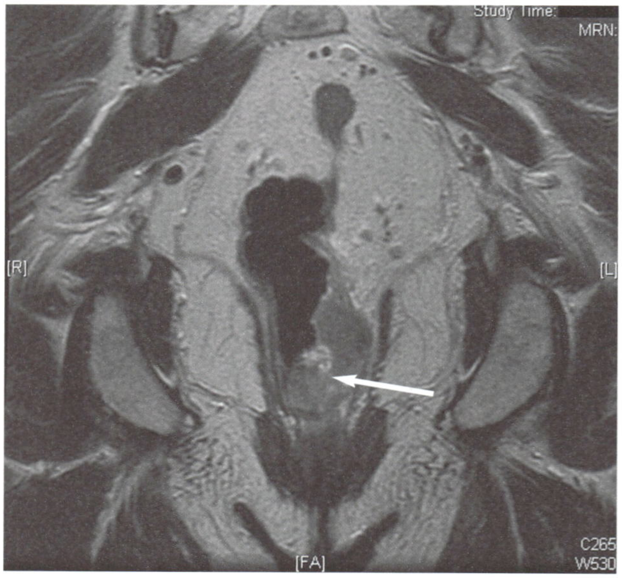

Figure 2. Pelvic MRI scan with a T3 rectal cancer. The arrow indicates that the T3 lesion has not broken out of the rectum. *Reproduced with permission from Dr M Tee, Consultant Radiologist, Leighton Hospital, Crewe, UK.*

What is a synchronous cancer?

Synchronous cancers are primary cancers which are detected at more than one site in the colorectum. At the time of first detection, about 2% of patients with colon and rectal cancers are found to have a second primary cancer.

Synchronous cancers are more frequently seen in patients who develop colorectal cancers in the setting of adenomatous polyposis coli, ulcerative colitis or HNPCC.

What is an abdominoperineal resection (APR)?

The standard surgical technique for the management of very low rectal cancers is an abdominoperineal resection.

This is a major operation which involves the complete excision of the rectum with the mesorectum (total mesorectal excision), anal sphincters and the entire anal canal. The operation is performed synchronously by two surgeons. Therefore, it is also referred to as synchronous combined abdomino-perineal excision of the rectum. At the end of the procedure, the perineal wound is closed and an end colostomy is erected in the left iliac fossa.

The laparoscopic-assisted abdominoperineal excision is being performed in some colorectal centres.

What is a total mesorectal excision (TME)?

One of the main challenges to a colorectal surgeon managing rectal cancers is the problem of local recurrence following surgery. The local recurrence of rectal cancer causes disabling symptoms which are difficult to treat.

Historically, the conventional technique of APR was associated with a high incidence of local recurrence of up to 15-45%.

Dr Quirk from Leeds first identified the high positive predictive value between the circumferential involvement of the rectum and the subsequent development of local recurrence of rectal cancer. The presence of tumour cells at the circumferential resection margin was identified by many other studies as one of the most important factors associated with the occurrence of local recurrence following surgery. The circumferential resection margin is now regarded as the best predictor of the adequacy of clearance of the mesorectum.

In 1982, Professor Heald from Basingstoke Hospital, UK, showed that the complete excision of the rectum, with its mesentery, can effectively reduce the incidence of local recurrence following rectal surgery. The operation was named a total mesorectal excision (TME) of the rectum.

The basic principle he advocated was to excise the rectum with the tumour *en bloc* to include the mesorectum (rectal mesentery) with its blood supply and lymphatic drainage. He adopted a fastidious approach to the technique and a 'specimen-oriented dissection' to achieve a complete mesorectal excision. The excised specimen *en bloc* has the appearance of a baby's bottom (Figure 3).

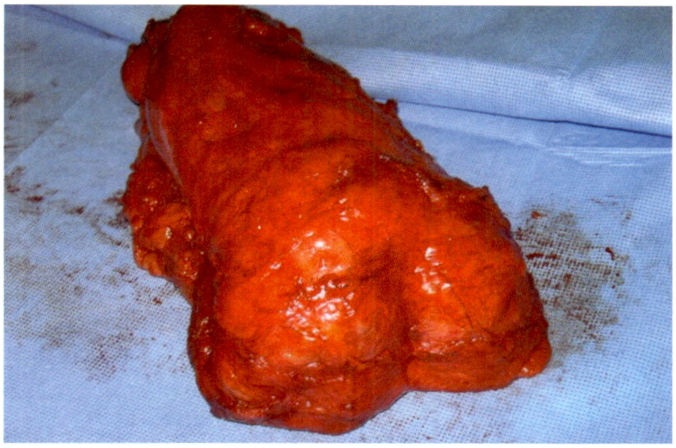

Figure 3. A total mesorectal excision (TME) specimen of a rectal cancer. ***Reproduced with permission from Mr CR Selvasekar, Colorectal Surgeon, Leighton Hospital, UK.***

Professor Heald published his first 100 cases of total mesorectal excision with a 0% 2-year local recurrence rate. His 5-year local recurrence was 4%. These impressive results were achieved without pre- or postoperative radiotherapy.

These results were reproduced by several studies. At present the total mesorectal excision is considered as the therapeutic gold standard for the treatment of rectal cancers in the middle and lower one third of the rectum.

Why is pre-operative radiotherapy considered in this patient?

Large meta-analyses and a prospective randomised multicentre trial (the Dutch TME trial) has shown that the combination of pre-operative radiotherapy and TME can improve the overall local recurrence rates and cancer-specific survival rates of rectal cancer (chemotherapy is now sometimes given as well as radiotherapy).

Why is a low anterior resection not considered in this patient?

The term 'anterior resection' is used to describe an anastomosis following the resection of rectal cancers found below 15cm from the dentate line. This patient has a rectal cancer 3cm from the dentate line. To adhere to the concept of TME and to achieve optimal distal margin clearance, it is likely that the colo-anal anastomosis of a low anterior resection would encroach on the sphincters.

There is evidence that especially in the elderly, a low anastomosis carries significant morbidity in terms of leak during the postoperative period, increased stool frequency and sphincter dysfunction. This patient has a locally advanced rectal cancer on pelvic MRI and unless the optimal clearance margins are achieved she is at a higher risk of developing local recurrences. The APR would give her the best chance of achieving a complete local clearance, to minimise the chance of local recurrence and improve survival. However, when anterior resections are performed appropriately there is a lower local recurrence rate than with APRs.

Clinical points

- Total mesorectal excision (TME) is considered as the therapeutic gold standard in the management of middle and lower one third rectal cancers.
- In general, T3 and T4 rectal cancers are considered for pre-operative radiotherapy.
- Pre-operative radiotherapy will downsize and downstage the tumour.
- There is evidence that neoadjuvant radiotherapy combined with TME offers the best outcome in terms of local recurrence and survival.
- The relative risks/benefits of short- and long-course radiotherapy are being assessed.
- There is no role for radiotherapy in the management of colon cancer.

Progress of the patient

- The patient undergoes an uneventful APR of the rectum after a long course of neoadjuvant radiotherapy. A TME dissection is carried out. All 21 nodes harvested are clear of tumour (Dukes' B).
- Histology is reviewed at the MDT meeting. The patient is seen by the oncologist and follow-up is planned.

Suggested reading

1. Kapiteijn E, Marijnen CAM, Nagtegaal ID, Putter H, Steup WH, Wiggers T, Rutten HJT, Pahlman L, Glimelius B, van Krieken JHJM, Leer JWH, van de Velde CJH, for the Dutch Colorectal Cancer Group. Preoperative radiotherapy combined with total mesorectal excision for resectable rectal cancer. *New Engl J Med* 2001; 345: 638-46.
2. Stockholm Colorectal Cancer Study Group. Randomized study on preoperative radiotherapy in rectal carcinoma. *Ann Surg Oncol* 1996; 3: 423-30.
3. Salerno G, Daniels I, Croxford M, Brown G, Heald RJ. Preoperative radiotherapy for rectal cancer. *J R Soc Med* 2004; 97(7): 361-62.
4. Guillem JG. As in fly fishing, 'matching the hatch' should govern the management of locally advanced rectal cancer. *Ann Surg* 2007; 246(5): 702-4.
5. Selvachandran SN, Cade D, *et al.* Prediction of colorectal cancer by a patient consultation questionnaire and scoring system: a prospective study. *The Lancet* 2002; 360; 278-83. PCQ web site: http://image.thelancet.com/extras/01art3336webquestionnaire.pdf.
6. Hodder RJ, *et al.* Pitfalls in the construction of cancer guidelines demonstrated by the analyses of colorectal referrals. *Ann R Coll Surg Eng* 2005; 87: 419-26.

Self-assessment

Q1
EMQ

Symptom combination:

a. Bright rectal bleeding during defecation.
b. Blood and mucous diarrhoea.
c. Left-sided abdominal colic, loose stools with mucus, a frequent desire for defecation, a sense of incomplete evacuation of faeces and weight loss.
d. Iron deficiency anaemia in the elderly.
e. A painful desire to defecate.
f. Severe anal pain at defecation.

Match the symptom combinations given above with the most likely pathology of the colorectum given below.

Most likely pathology:

1. Cancer in the rectum.
2. Caecal cancer.
3. Haemorrhoids.
4. Acute anal fissure.
5. Ulcerative colitis.

Q2
SBA

An 85-year-old women who has had her colonic polyps excised 10 years ago was lost to follow-up. She now presents with iron deficiency anaemia. She has not been on NSAID treatment and she is a non-alcoholic. She has no alteration of bowels. Two of the three faecal occult blood samples are positive.

What is the most likely pathology responsible for her occult blood loss?

a. Oesophageal varices.
b. Chronic peptic ulcer disease.
c. Right colon cancer.
d. Haemorrhoids.
e. Diverticular disease.

Q3
SBA

A 78-year-old man is found to have a poorly differentiated rectal cancer at 5cm from the anal verge. An MRI shows that the lesion is a T4 tumour. The colonoscopy shows that the lesion is 4cm in length involving 60% of the circumference. A CT scan shows no metastatic disease.

What is the most appropriate next step in the management of this patient?

a. Radiotherapy.
b. Low anterior resection and defunctioning ileostomy.
c. Neoadjuvant radiotherapy followed by abdomino-perineal resection.
d. Hartmann's procedure.
e. Chemotherapy.

Q4
True/False

a. MRI is a better tool than a CT scan to assess the local spread of rectal cancer.
b. MRI is associated with a radiation hazard.
c. MRI cannot be performed in patients with total hip replacements.
d. Transrectal ultrasound is a tool to assess the local extension of rectal cancer.
e. Tissue samples of mesorectal lymph nodes may be obtained during transrectal ultrasound.

Q5
True/False

Synchronous cancers of the colorectum:

a. Are primary cancers which are detected in more than one site in the colorectum.
b. Are seen in about 2% of patients with colon and rectal cancers.
c. Are more frequently seen in patients who develop colorectal cancers in the setting of ulcerative colitis.

d. Are more likely to be seen in patients with genetic defects involving the DNA repair system.
e. If found in the left and right colon in a middle-aged patient, a total colectomy should be considered as the definitive treatment.

Q6
True/False

Local recurrence following surgery for rectal cancer:

a. Is rare following abdominoperineal resection.
b. Is uncommon following total mesorectal excision.
c. Is more frequent if the tumour perforates during excision.
d. Can be minimised with neoadjuvant radiotherapy.
e. Is more frequent when the circumferential resection margin is involved.

Q7
True/False

a. The resection of rectal cancers below 15cm from the dentate line and primary anastomosis is called an anterior resection.
b. The lower the anastomosis in an anterior resection, the higher the morbidity.
c. Pre-operative radiotherapy will downsize and downstage the rectal cancer.
d. Neoadjuvant radiotherapy and TME offers the best outcome in terms of local recurrence and survival.
e. There is no role for radiotherapy in the management of colon cancer.

Answers overleaf

Self-assessment answers

Q1 1. (c), 2. (d), 3. (a), 4. (f), 5. (e).

Q2 (c).

Q3 (c).

Explanatory notes

This male patient has a locally advanced, partially obstructing, poorly differentiated low rectal cancer.

The benefits of low anterior resection should be weighted against significant morbidity related to increased stool frequency, sphincter dysfunction and the risk of incomplete tumour clearance in an elderly male. Studies have shown that the combination of pre-operative radiotherapy and TME can improve the overall local recurrence rates and cancer-specific survival rates of rectal cancer.

Q4 a. (T), b. (F), c. (T), d. (T), e. (T).

Q5 a. (T), b. (T), c. (T), d. (T), e. (T).

Q6 a. (F), b. (T), c. (T), d. (T), e. (T).

Q7 a. (T), b. (T), c. (T), d. (T), e. (T).

Chapter 12

Anal fissures, suppuration, sinuses, fistulae and piles

Learning objectives

- To learn the differential diagnosis and management of painful anal conditions.
- To understand the causes and pathogenesis of piles, fissures, peri-anal suppurations, sinuses and fistulae.
- To appreciate the relationship between piles and fissures.
- To learn the principles of treatment of piles.

Case scenario

A 30-year-old bank executive presents with a 1-week history of anal pain. The pain gets worse during and after defecation. On a few occasions he has seen a streak of bright red blood on the toilet paper and a few drops of blood in the toilet. He had a similar episode about 2 months ago that responded to laxatives. He is under stress, working late hours to meet targets.

He has no other comorbid conditions. The general examination is unremarkable.

The anal examination reveals a swollen anal skin tag in the posterior midline at the anal verge. There is no swelling, erythema or ulceration in the per-anal region but attempted separation of the anal canal is met with severe pain and a tear is visible in the posterior midline of the anal canal. Digital rectal examination is not possible. His haematological parameters are normal.

The most likely clinical diagnosis: an acute posterior anal fissure.

Acute posterior anal fissure is the most common cause of acute anal pain. A fissure is a tear or a split. The tear usually extends to the anal verge. The posterior midline is the commonest site of a tear; approximately 90% of all anal fissures occur in the posterior midline. The most characteristic symptom of an acute anal fissure is the intense pain associated with and after defecation. The fissures may bleed.

The tear occurs due to trauma during the passage of a hard stool. Many patients with acute anal fissures are constipated. Many young patients are also found to have high anal canal pressures which interfere with the passage of a hard stool mass. An attempted passage of a dry stool mass through a fissure increases the anal sphincter tone further, because the sphincter goes into spasm due to pain.

Patients are anxious to open their bowels because of severe pain. A positive vicious circle develops which consists of pain, constipation, trauma and sphincter spasm.

Repeated episodes of acute fissures can result in the formation of deep chronic anal fissures.

If recurrent fissures and infection are present, Crohn's disease needs to be excluded. The anal fissures in Crohn's disease often do not occur in the midline.

Deep chronic anal fissures may mimic anal cancer.

Clinical points

- Anal fissure:
  - the most common cause of acute anal pain;
  - the most common site is the posterior midline;
  - when found away from the midline and recurrent with sepsis, Crohn's disease needs to be excluded.

Is there a relationship between piles and fissures?

It is not uncommon for patients with anal fissures to develop haemorrhoids or piles.

Piles are submucosal cushions that constitute the normal anatomy of the anal canal. They function as the final closure mechanism of the anal canal; like a washer of a tap that stops the last few drops of water after closure. When these normal cushions get exposed to high anal canal pressures over a period of time, due to straining as a result of constipation and/or high anal canal pressures from an increase in resting anal sphincter tone, they become symptomatic.

The cushions become large as they undergo hypertrophy. They become loose from their attachment from the wall of the anal canal and start prolapsing out during the passage of a stool mass. The passage of a dry stool under pressure causes erosion of the cushions which begin to bleed. The chronic irritation causes hyperplasia of the mucous glands which produce mucus discharge and cause anal itching. Longstanding hypertrophy leads to permanent prolapse of large pile masses which may undergo thrombosis and strangulation. Only then do piles become painful. Strangulated haemorrhoids may get infected.

The five symptoms, swelling, bleeding, itching, mucous discharge and pain, are interpreted by the patient as 'piles'.

As the pile begins to prolapse, part of the pile lies in the anal canal and the remainder presents out as a lump which is easily palpable and visible at the anus. The proximal part of this lump is lined by stratified squamous epithelium of the anal canal and the remainder is lined by squamous epithelium of the skin. The internal part of the lump is referred to as the internal haemorrhoid and the external part is loosely referred to as the external haemorrhoid. In general, what is most common is the combination of the two, the so called intero-external haemorrhoid.

Based on the size of the lump, piles can be classified into four stages:

- Grade I. The patient presents with bleeding per rectum and proctoscopic examination reveals piles.
- Grade II. The patient complains of the appearance of a lump during defecation which reduces spontaneously after the act.
- Grade III. There is a lump which appears during defecation but will not reduce until the patient manually reduces it.
- Grade IV. A permanent prolapse.

Anal skin tags are not uncommon in mothers after child birth. They are not considered as true haemorrhoids. No treatment is indicated unless they cause symptoms such as irritation and itching due to trapping of faecal matter.

Progress of the patient

- The patient is informed of the following:
  - the sequence of events that leads to a fissure to help his understanding on how to break the vicious cycle;
  - the majority will heal without any surgical treatment;
  - to increase the intake of liquids to reduce the dryness of the stool;
  - to apply glyceryl trinitrate (GTN) ointment to the anal margin;
  - 50% patients will get headaches with GTN ointment;
  - to have a stool softener during the initial period and then a stool bulking agent to form a bulky stool that facilitates the smooth passage.

The local application of glyceryl trinitrate (GTN) is shown to be beneficial in the treatment of acute anal fissures. Nitric oxide is an important inhibitory neurotransmitter which causes relaxation of the internal anal sphincter. GTN is an exogenous nitric oxide donor.

An alternative to GTN is topical diltiazem, a calcium channel blocker, which has shown to be associated with less adverse effects including headache in at least one randomised controlled trial.

Botulinum toxin (Botox) injection is another alternative. It acts by relaxing the external anal sphincter. It is expensive, however.

Most primary care physicians prescribe a local anaesthetic gel as the initial treatment.

Progress of the patient

- The patient responds to local application of GTN.
- He is referred by the primary care physician after 6 months with recurrence of the pain.
- Examination reveals a deep chronic fissure which could not be assessed because of pain.
- He has been absent from work for 1 week because of the pain, and the local anaesthetic gel that the primary care physician has prescribed has not worked.
- He is admitted for examination under anaesthesia (EUA) and anal sphincterotomy.

What are the other treatment options for anal fissures?

Manual dilatation of the anus was the conventional treatment. The principle behind this approach was to relieve the anal sphincter tone. This is not favoured by many because of the suboptimal results due to under-dilatation and complications that result from over-dilatation of the anal canal. Permanent incontinence has been reported.

The most favoured approach is a partial controlled lateral internal sphincterotomy.

Progress of the patient

- The EUA shows a chronic posterior anal fissure and a tight anal sphincter.
- There is no evidence of anal suppuration, an anal fistula or an anal sinus. Flexible sigmoidoscopy shows no other abnormalities except minor haemorrhoids.

What is the next step?

- He undergoes a partial controlled lateral internal sphincterotomy. This patient has a recurrent posterior anal fissure which is chronic. Sphincterotomy is the recommended treatment at this stage.

What is a sphincterotomy?

Sphincterotomy is division of the sphincter. In the anal canal there are two sphincters: the internal anal sphincter and the external anal sphincter. It is like one flower pot inside the other, the internal sphincter being the inner flower pot. The space between the two is called the inter-sphincteric plane. The internal sphincter is responsible for the resting anal pressure and is involuntary. The external sphincter is used for voluntary control. It is responsible for the squeeze pressure.

The operation of sphincterotomy involves partial division of the internal sphincter laterally. The external sphincter is not divided.

The tone of the internal anal sphincter, external anal sphincter and anorectal ring contributes to maintain continence. The anorectal ring is formed by some fibres of the internal sphincter, deep fibres of the external sphincter and the puborectalis muscle, which is the medial part of the levator ani muscle. Therefore, a partial division of the internal anal sphincter will relieve the anal canal pressures and facilitate healing of the fissure but will not cause any significant continence problems. The site of division is in the lateral position of the anal canal, at the 3 or 9 o'clock position in a controlled fashion. This is why it is called partial controlled lateral internal sphincterotomy.

Progress of the patient

- Eight weeks after surgery the patient reports an excellent response to treatment. Digital rectal examination reveals that the fissure is almost completely healed. He also reports a slight inability to 'control wind' which he experienced for a few weeks following surgery. This symptom has since resolved.
- The patient is reminded on the importance of a high intake of liquids and fibre and he is discharged under the care of the primary care physician.

Flatus incontinence is reported by some patients. Patients should be warned of this symptom during the consenting process. This usually resolves as seen in this patient.

What are the principles of treatment for haemorrhoids?

Piles are treated only when they are symptomatic with minimum possible intervention on a physiological basis. The lifestyle changes to address the causation of piles, to include an increase in fluid and high fibre intake, are important to prevent recurrence.

It is mandatory to exclude cancer of the rectum and anal canal before diagnosing piles as the sole cause of anorectal symptoms.

Treatment of the cause

Constipation and high anal sphincter tone are two key factors. A simple lifestyle change which includes a high fibre diet and increased intake of fluid is mandatory to the long-term outcome of any interventional treatment which may follow.

Most fluid is absorbed in the small bowel and by the large bowel, the rest is absorbed by fibre. Fibre constitutes cellulose, hemi-cellulose and pectin. The fibres we eat reach the large bowel unchanged, because the human digestive system has no enzymes to digest fibre.

The fluid absorbed by fibre increases the bulkiness of the stool and reduces its dryness. Therefore, an increase in fluid and fibre will increase the bulk of the stool mass which facilitates easy passage.

Symptomatic treatment

Uncomplicated haemorrhoids usually do not cause pain. The symptoms which require treatment are bleeding and prolapse.

Two commonly used methods to treat bleeding are injection sclerotherapy with oily phenol and the application of rubber bands to the base of the haemorrhoid. These are performed on an outpatient basis.

Sclerotherapy causes sclerosis or fibrosis which makes piles more adherent to the wall of the anal canal.

The bands occlude the blood flow and the pile becomes ischaemic. Part of the pile mass then sloughs off. This reduces the size and the resultant scar becomes adherent to the wall.

The present evidence suggests that the outcome of banding is superior to sclerotherapy.

Excisional surgery is indicted for large prolapsing haemorrhoids after failed banding, especially in those with a significant external component.

Elderly patients with lax anal sphincters and large pile masses may need excisional surgery. Postoperative pain and strictures are the main disadvantages of this approach.

Modern stapling devices are available. Stapled haemorrhoidectomy is shown to be associated with reduced postoperative pain.

Exclusion of cancer

All five previously mentioned clinical features of piles can also be caused by cancer of the anal canal or rectum. Haemorrhoids are extremely common. Cancers are uncommon. Cancers and piles often coexist.

Piles can also be the result of cancer when the invasion causes interference with the venous drainage that makes the piles swell.

Haemorrhoids, however, do not predispose to cancer. Therefore, it is mandatory to exclude cancer as the cause of bleeding, before diagnosing piles as the cause. This is best done with a flexible sigmoidoscope.

Clinical points

- Treatment of piles:
  - endoscopic or surgical treatment is indicated for piles only when they produce significant symptoms.
  - it is mandatory to exclude cancer as the cause of 'symptoms of piles' before commencing treatment for piles.

What are the other conditions that can cause anal pain?

- Peri-anal haematoma. A peri-anal haematoma presents as an acutely painful swelling at the anal margin. It will regress spontaneously but a haematoma is best evacuated at an early stage under local or general anaesthesia.
- Thrombosed haemorrhoids.
- Anal suppuration (peri-anal abscesses, infected anal sinuses or fistulae [Figures 1 and 2]).
- Proctalgia fugax. A spasmodic-type severe anal pain commonly affecting females which tends to regress spontaneously.

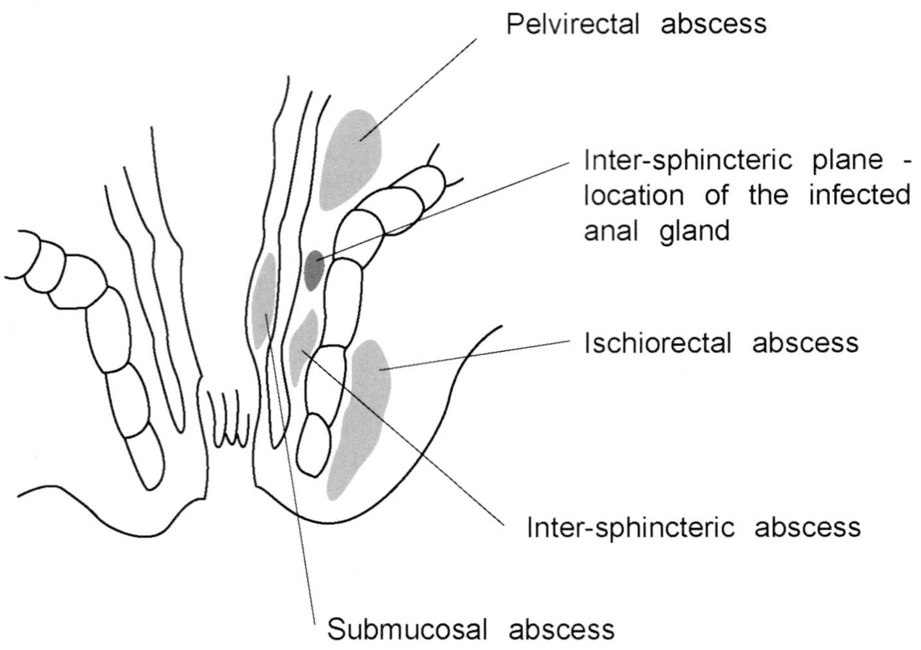

Figure 1. Locations of anal suppuration.

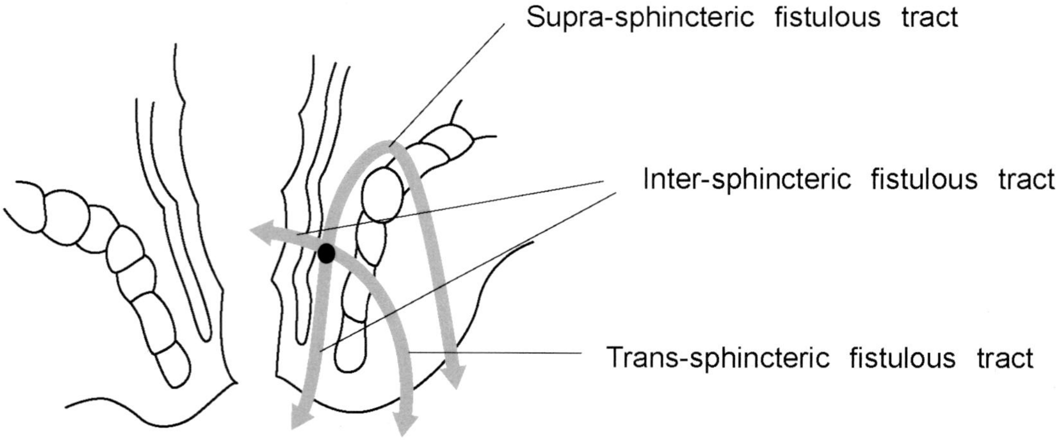

Figure 2. Diagrammatic representation of peri-anal fistulae.

What is the relationship between anal suppuration, an anal sinus and an anal fistula?

Understanding the pathogenesis of suppurative lesions around the anus is fundamental to appreciate this relationship.

Infection in the anal canal is the main initiating event. The initial site of infection is the anal glands. The anal glands are found between the internal and external sphincter, in the inter-sphincteric plane. They pass through the internal sphincter and open into anal crypts in the anal canal. Blockage of the duct of the anal gland causes accumulation of its contents that becomes infected. A small abscess develops in the inter-sphincteric plane. The collection of pus commonly drains downwards in the inter-sphincteric plane along the line of least resistance and presents as an acutely tender swelling at the anal verge.

Once the abscess is drained, the event may regress completely. However, if the chronic infection continues, the tract will persist and will become lined by granulation tissue. An inter-sphincteric sinus is thus formed.

If the infected anal gland site forms a tract that drains through the internal sphincter into the anal canal, the inter-sphincteric sinus becomes an inter-sphincteric fistula. A fistula is a tract lined by granulation tissue that connects two epithelial lined surfaces. Depending on the site of entry into the anal canal, it is referred to as a low or high fistula.

With different drainage pathways of peri-anal abscesses, fistulae such as trans-sphincteric, supra-sphincteric and extra-sphincteric fistulae may develop. These are uncommon.

The principle of treatment of peri-anal sinuses and fistulae is to drain the infected site, eradicate the underlying infected gland and tract by excising it as completely as possible and preserve the sphincter function.

Suggested reading

1. Bielecki K, Kolodziejczak M. A prospective randomized trial of diltiazem and glyceryltrinitrate ointment in the treatment of chronic anal fissure. *Colorectal Disease* 2003; 5: 256-7.
2. Parks AG, Hardcastle JD, Gordon P. A classification of fistula-in-ano. *Br J Surg* 1976; 63: 1-12.
3. Parks AG, Stitz RW. The treatment of high fistula-in-ano. *Dis Colon Rectum* 1976; 19: 487-99.
4. Aluwihare APR. Finding the source of a fistula. *Colorectal Disease* 2005; 7: 528-9.

Self-assessment

Q1
EMQ

a. Crohn's disease.
b. Acute anal fissure.
c. Anal fistula.
d. Anal haematoma.
e. Haemorrhoids.

Select the most likely clinical diagnosis from the conditions mentioned above for the clinical presentation described below.

1. Discharging site in the peri-anal region.
2. Painful swelling at the anal verge.
3. Painless intermittent fresh bleeding PR.
4. Painful bleeding PR.
5. Multiple anal sinuses and fissures.

Q2
EMQ

a. Anal dilatation.
b. Partial controlled lateral internal sphincterotomy.
c. Botulin toxin injection.
d. GTN ointment.
e. Rubber band ligation.
f. Topical antibiotics.
g. None of above.
h. Injection of oily phenol.

Select the most appropriate treatment options or statements from above for the clinical presentations described below.

1. First episode of acute anal fissure.
2. Recurrent painful anal fissure.
3. Bleeding internal haemorrhoids.
4. Anal fistula.

Q3
SBA

What is the most appropriate next step in the management of a patient who presents with chronic recurrent painful anal fissures and peri-anal sepsis?

a. Proctoscopy, rectal biopsy.
b. Colonoscopy.
c. Examination under anaesthesia (EUA).
d. EUA, sigmoidoscopy and rectal biopsy.
e. EUA and colonoscopy.

Q4
True/False

Haemorrhoids:

a. Are submucosal cushions.
b. Are the most common cause of anal pain.
c. Predispose to cancer.
d. Symptoms can mimic cancer.
e. Bleed often and resolve spontaneously.

Q5
True/False

a. The majority of patients with symptomatic haemorrhoids need surgical excision.
b. The majority of patients with acute anal fissure need surgical treatment.
c. The majority of patients with anal fistulae need surgical treatment.
d. Insertion of a seton is recognised treatment for a high anal fistula.
e. A defunctioning colostomy is indicated for major rectal trauma.

Answers overleaf

Self-assessment answers

Q1 1. (c), 2. (d), 3. (e), 4. (b), 5. (a).

Q2 1. (d), 2. (b), 3. (e), 4. (g).

Q3 (d). Anorectal Crohn's disease needs to be excluded.

Q4 a. (T), b. (F), c. (F), d. (T), e. (T).

Q5 a. (F), b. (F), c. (T), d. (T), e. (T).

Chapter 13

Acute intestinal obstruction

Learning objectives

- To learn the clinical and radiological features of acute small bowel obstruction.
- To recollect the pathophysiology of intestinal obstruction.
- To appreciate the importance of early recognition of impending strangulation.
- To learn the process of clinical judgment and decision making with regards to management.
- To understand the indications, value and limitations of a contrast CT scan in the management of acute intestinal obstruction.

Case scenario

A 45-year-old male presents with colicky abdominal pain of 24 hours' duration. The symptoms began about an hour after lunch on the previous day. It improved after vomiting but the pain returned in about an hour. Since then he has been experiencing intermittent central abdominal colic. Soon after the onset of pain, he had a bowel motion but has not passed stools or flatus since that time. He denies any similar episodes. A year ago he had undergone a laparotomy for a stab injury to his abdomen.

On examination, his temperature is 100°F, pulse rate is 102/minute and RR is 22/minute. The abdomen is distended with a well healed midline scar. The abdomen is generally tender but there is no evidence of peritonitis or masses. The bowel sounds are hyperactive with occasional high pitched rushes and tinkling sounds. No external herniae are identified. Rectal examination reveals no masses and an empty rectum.

The results of the investigations are:

- White cell count - 12,000/mm^3 with 84% neutrophils and 10% lymphocytes.
- Hb 14g/dL.
- S amylase 30U/L.

The most likely clinical diagnosis: acute intestinal obstruction.

Central colicky abdominal pain, abdominal distension, nausea, vomiting and absolute constipation are the cardinal clinical features of acute mechanical intestinal obstruction.

The level of obstruction has a bearing on the clinical picture. For example, vomiting will appear early in high small bowel obstruction but the distension will be less marked. In distal ileal obstruction the vomiting will be a later feature and the distension will be more prominent.

Central colicky abdominal pain is usually due to mechanical obstruction of the small intestine or the proximal colon (embryological midgut). This is caused by referred pain transmitted via the autonomic nervous system in association with the superior mesenteric artery.

It is very likely that this patient has acute mechanical small bowel obstruction.

A history of a previous laparotomy and the absence of an obstructing external hernia indicate that the most likely cause for the acute small bowel obstruction is postoperative adhesions.

In general, about 50% of acute small bowel obstructions are due to postoperative adhesions. About 15% are caused by external or internal herniae.

Acute large bowel obstruction due to postoperative adhesions usually does not occur because, unlike the small bowel which easily gets kinked on its loose mesentery, the large bowel is mostly retroperitoneal.

Clinical points

- Central colicky abdominal pain, abdominal distension, nausea, vomiting and absolute constipation to faeces and flatus are the cardinal clinical features of acute mechanical intestinal obstruction.
- Central colicky abdominal pain is usually due to mechanical obstruction of the small intestine or the proximal colon.

However, in some patients, the clinical picture may not be very clear.

In general, the most likely cause of acute intestinal obstruction will depend upon:

- The age of the patient.
- The onset and duration of symptoms.
- Whether the patient has had an abdominal operation or not.
- A previous history suggestive of an intestinal pathology such as Crohn's disease, diverticular disease or carcinoma.
- A previous history of surgery for bowel cancer.

Certain physical and radiological signs may give clues.

A meticulous examination may reveal visible small bowel loops on the anterior abdominal wall which support the diagnosis of small bowel obstruction, in a thin patient.

A small femoral hernia with a loop of small bowel causing acute small bowel obstruction may not be easily detectable in an obese female unless it is looked for, because a non-tender femoral hernia may be hidden in the fat of the groin.

An elderly patient presenting with abdominal pain of sudden onset with severe distension and a tympanic abdomen raises the possibility of an acute sigmoid volvulus which can be confirmed with a supine abdominal X-ray.

Clinical points

- In the absence of an obstructing external hernia, postoperative adhesions are the most likely cause of obstruction in a patient who presents with intestinal obstruction with a past history of abdominal surgery.
- Acute large bowel obstruction due to adhesions does not usually occur.

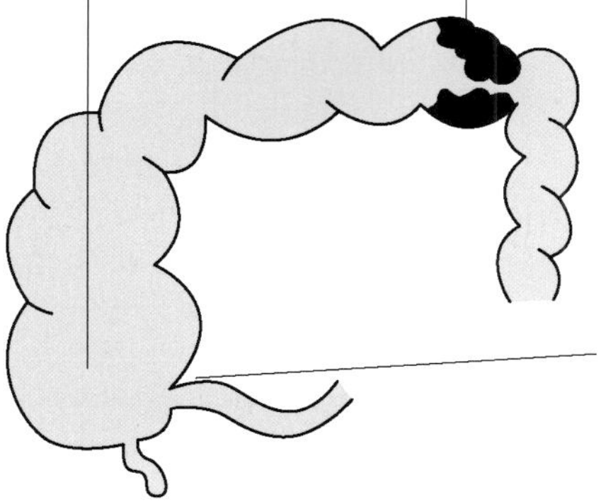

Figure 1. Diagrammatic representation of a closed loop obstruction.

In a patient presenting with features of intestinal obstruction, the finding of a distended caecum in the right iliac fossa on abdominal X-ray with localised tenderness over the caecum raises the possibility of a closed loop obstruction with impending caecal perforation.

Closed loop obstruction (Figure 1) occurs in patients with an obstructing colon cancer with a competent ileocaecal valve. The segment of bowel between the site of obstruction and ileocaecal valve becomes a 'closed loop'. This segment becomes progressively distended with fluid and air produced by the gas-forming organisms. The competent ileocaecal valve acts as a one-way valve and therefore the large bowel cannot deflate to the small bowel. The distended segment of the bowel soon becomes ischaemic and perforates resulting in faecal peritonitis. This condition carries a high mortality.

Localised tenderness in the left iliac fossa may suggest an inflammatory diverticular mass or an abscess which may be associated with a diverticular stricture. Crohn's disease, tuberculous strictures of the small bowel or colon and gallstone ileus are other uncommon causes to be considered in adults presenting with acute small bowel obstruction. Crohn's disease is less common in Asia and TB strictures are rare in the western hemisphere.

In the elderly and in patients with atrial fibrillation, mesenteric ischaemia may present with a picture of acute intestinal obstruction.

Obstruction in a neonate, an infant or in a young child is most likely the result of a hernia, malrotation, meconium ileus, Meckel's diverticulum, intussusception or intestinal atresia.

What is the next step?

- A supine abdominal X-ray film is obtained.

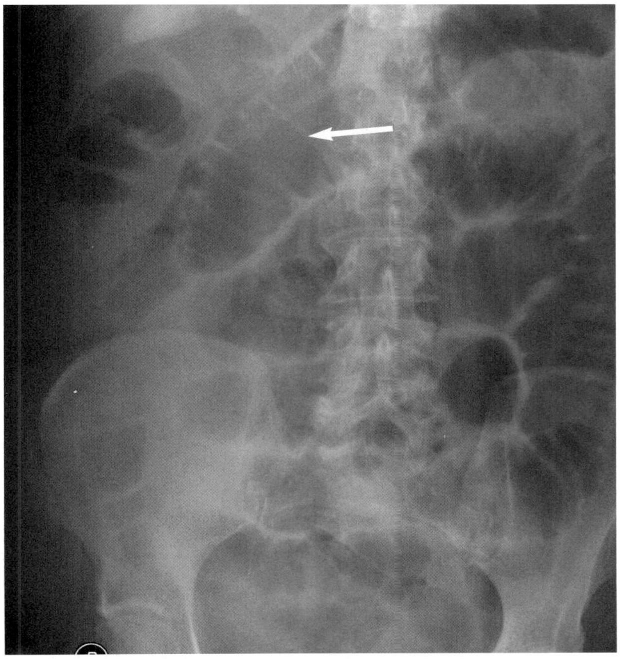

Figure 2. A supine abdominal X-ray of an acute small bowel obstruction. Transverse bands which traverse across the bowel are indicated by the white arrow. ***Reproduced with permission from Dr M Tee, Consultant Radiologist, Leighton Hospital, Crewe, UK.***

What are the characteristic features seen in this X-ray?

- The bowel loops are placed more centrally. Small bowel is in the centre of the abdomen.
- Transverse bands which traverse across the bowel (valvulae conniventes) are seen (Figure 2). This is a feature to recognise the small bowel.
- The diameter of some of the small bowel loops is more than 5cm, which indicates that there is evidence of pathological dilatation of the small bowel.

How do the radiological features differ in acute large bowel obstruction?

In acute large bowel obstruction:

- The dilated bowel is seen mostly in the periphery of the film.
- The bands (haustrae) incompletely traverse the bowel (Figure 3).
- Dilatation of the large bowel >8cm is considered as pathological.
- Dilatation of the caecum >10cm suggests impending rupture.

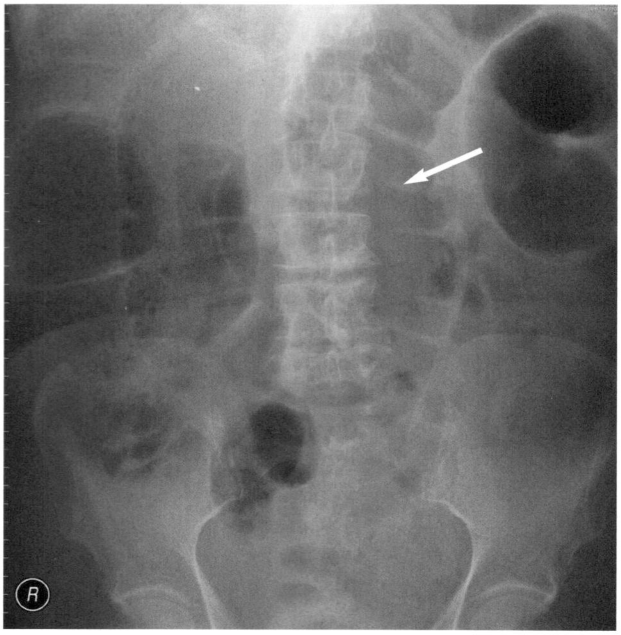

Figure 3. A supine abdominal X-ray of an acute large bowel obstruction. Haustrae incompletely traverse the bowel (white arrow). ***Reproduced with permission from Dr M Tee, Consultant Radiologist, Leighton Hospital, Crewe, UK.***

What is the place for an erect abdominal X-ray?

In the past, erect and supine abdominal X-rays were routinely performed when intestinal obstruction was suspected. But many specialised GI centres have stopped performing erect films as little extra information is gained from them. However, it may be useful in early bowel obstruction, when isolated fluid levels may be evident.

What is the next step?

- Conservative management is commenced.
- Baseline bloods (FBC, renal and liver profile, blood grouping) are obtained.
- A nasogastric tube is placed to decompress the stomach.
- Fluid resuscitation is commenced with N saline.
- The patient is catheterised to monitor urine output and assess the response to fluid resuscitation.
- Low-molecular-weight heparin is given subcutaneously for deep vein thrombosis (DVT) prophylaxis.
- Repeated clinical assessment is performed with a special emphasis on:
  - change in the pattern of symptoms;
  - change in the physical signs;
  - general condition;
  - pulse chart;
  - blood pressure chart;
  - temperature chart.

Most patients with acute small bowel obstruction due to adhesions will respond to conservative management. These are the patients who have no evidence suggestive of bowel ischaemia such as constant pain, fever, peritoneal signs or leucocytosis. They are classified as simple mechanical obstruction. The obstructed bowel deflates when the bowel is given a short period of rest.

Non-operative treatment is frequently successful in patients with simple mechanical small bowel obstruction due to adhesions. However, some may develop complications when progressive obstruction leads to strangulation as the blood supply to the segment becomes occluded. Ischaemia to the affected segment of bowel leads to necrosis, gangrene, perforation and peritonitis. Therefore, non-operative treatment is clearly inappropriate for patients with evidence of impending or existing bowel ischaemia.

The 'red flag' features which suggest impending ischaemia to a segment of bowel in patients with acute small bowel obstruction due to adhesions are:

- Deteriorating general condition.
- Change in the pattern of pain from colicky type to constant.
- Rising temperature - see the temperature chart.
- Rising pulse rate - see the pulse chart.
- General diffuse vague tenderness becoming localised and increased in severity with evidence of peritoneal irritation such as an inability to move or cough without a sharp increase in pain.

Mechanical obstruction of the small bowel will cause accumulation of fluid inside the distended bowel lumen and also in the bowel wall. This leads to depletion of the intravascular fluid volume and a decrease in perfusion to all other organs.

Early recognition and restoration of the intravascular volume to re-establish organ perfusion is important prior to operative treatment because the induction of general anesthesia in a volume-depleted patient may result in profound hypotension and complications including renal failure.

In health, the amount of fluid entering and passing through the small bowel may be up to 9 litres per day (Table 1).

Table 1. Fluid entering small intestine per 24 hours.

- Diet - 2000-2500ml.
- Saliva - 500ml.
- Gastric juice - 1500-3000ml.
- Pancreatic juice - 750-1500ml.
- Bile - 750-1500ml.
- Total - 5500-9000ml.

Clinical points

- The important aspects of management are early diagnosis, restoration of circulatory volume to re-establish organ perfusion and clinical judgment to discontinue conservative treatment.

Progress of the patient

- The patient is re-assessed after 24 hours of admission.
- The patient remains unwell. The abdominal colic has become more frequent since admission and now he complains of persistent pain. He has not passed flatus or faeces.
- Pulse chart - persistent tachycardia 122 beats/minute.
- BP chart - no change.
- Temperature chart - a spike of temperature 100.9°F.
- Fluid balance chart:
  - total intake = 4,850ml (N saline and Hartmann's solution);
  - total output = 4,750ml;
  - nasogastric tube output = 3000ml;
  - urine output = 1750ml - hourly urine output has dropped to 20ml/hr during the last 2 hours.

Progress of the patient

- Abdominal examination:
  - distended;
  - bowel sounds are present but less active;
  - localised tenderness to the left of the midline abdominal scar.
- WCC 16,000mm^3.
- Serum sodium (Na) 130mml/L.
- Serum potassium (K) 3.1mmol/L.
- Blood urea 8mmol/L.
- The patient is developing evidence of impending bowel ischaemia and increasing third space loss.
- A central line is inserted to measure the CVP. The patient's CVP is +2.
- Fluid resuscitation is increased.
- The electrolyte deficit is corrected.
- The decision is made to perform an exploratory laparotomy.

The key issues which influence clinical judgment are:

- Change in the pain pattern from colicky to persistent.
- Deteriorating general condition.
- Pyrexia.
- Tachycardia.
- Localised tenderness.
- Rising white cell count.

The change in the pain pattern from colicky to persistent is a major concern. Persistent pain may be due to two reasons. It may be due to severe bowel distension (which produces localised venous congestion, decreased bowel perfusion and eventually necrosis and gangrene) or bowel ischaemia secondary to strangulation of the bowel. The strangulation means that a segment of the bowel has run short of its blood supply. This is either due to twisting of its mesentery secondary to the severe distension or the mesentery with its blood vessels has become compressed at the neck of an external (inguinal or femoral) hernia or internal hernia.

Localised tenderness is also a major concern. Small bowel distension produces non-specific tenderness which is poorly localised. But when bowel ischaemia sets in, it causes focal peritoneal signs such as localised tenderness and guarding over the affected bowel. Fever, tachycardia and rising white cell count are the other warning features of impending ischaemia.

Progress of the patient

- A broad-spectrum antibiotic (e.g. cefuroxime or ciprofloxacin) together with metronidazole 500mg are administered at induction.
- At laparotomy, a distended segment of the ileum which is 9cm in length is found about 12cm from the ileocaecal junction. The adhesions are divided and the segment of bowel is released. The bowel appears viable after releasing the adhesions. The distended proximal small bowel is gently decompressed by 'milking' the contents towards the nasogastric tube while the segment of the released bowel is packed with a large gauze swab soaked with warm saline.
- The anaesthetist increases the oxygen delivery to the patient.
- After milking the contents of the proximal bowel, the affected segment is re-examined for signs of viability. The segment now appears pink and the mesenteric arterial pulsations are becoming more evident. The remaining abdominal viscera are inspected. More adhesions are divided. No other abnormalities are found.

Progress of the patient

- During the postoperative period the patient is given low-molecular-weight heparin subcutaneously daily for DVT prophylaxis.
- Oral fluids are commenced on the second postoperative day as the patient sensed the passage of flatus.
- A soft diet is commenced on the third postoperative day.

What is the role of contrast CT in the management of acute intestinal obstruction?

A contrast CT scan is indicated if the clinical picture is confusing, complicated or if the plain films are unhelpful.

There is a tendency at present to use contrast CT scans more frequently in acute settings.

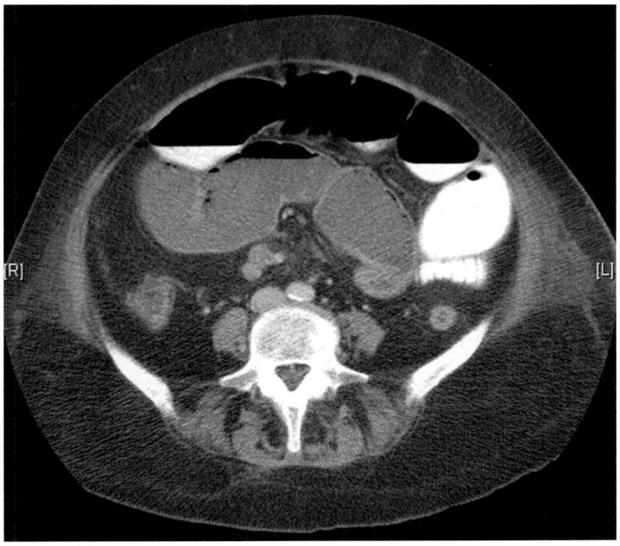

Figure 4. A contrast CT film of an acute small bowel obstruction. ***Reproduced with permission from Dr M Tee, Consultant Radiologist, Leighton Hospital, Crewe, UK.***

Contrast CT scans may demonstrate the following:

- Level of the obstruction.
- Cause of the obstruction.
- Degree of obstruction.
- Viability of the affected bowel.

A CT scan is also useful for detecting bowel masses, peritoneal thickenings and liver lesions (Figure 4).

The main limitation is the need to administer contrast into the bowel which can contribute to vomiting and aspiration in elderly patients.

Progress of the patient

- The patient is discharged on the eighth postoperative day on a normal diet.
- During the first clinic visit he appears to be progressing well. He seeks reassurance that this will not happen again, but is informed that it is not possible to give such a reassurance. However, the majority of patients who have a tendency to develop adhesions cope well. He is advised to avoid diets with excessive fibre and to make sure that he has a good liquid intake.

Suggested reading

1. Miller G, Boman J, Shrier I, Gordon PH. Natural history of patients with adhesive small bowel obstruction. *Br J Surg* 2000; 87 (9): 1240-7.
2. Cox MR, Gunn IF, Eastman MC, Hunt RF, Heinz AW. The safety and duration of non-operative treatment for adhesive small bowel obstruction. *Aust NZ J Surg* 1993; 63(5): 367-71.

Self-assessment

Q1
EMQ

a. Closed loop obstruction.
b. Peritonitis.
c. Small bowel obstruction due to adhesions.
d. Leaking abdominal aortic aneurysm.

Select the most likely clinical diagnosis from the conditions mentioned above for the case scenarios described below.

1. A 75-year-old man presents with altered bowels and a distended abdomen. There is tenderness over the caecum. A distended caecum shows up on plain X-ray.
2. A 35-year-year old man presents with a history of laparotomy for a stab injury 8 months ago, abdominal pain, distension and absolute constipation of 3 days' duration, and a reducible inguinal hernia.
3. An 80-year-old female who has collapsed at home presents with abdominal pain of 1 week's duration. She is pyrexial, with lower abdominal tenderness and has a BP of 100/60mm Hg.
4. A 76-year-old male has collapsed at home, with severe abdominal and back pain of sudden onset. He is obese, sweaty and has some abdominal distension. His BP is 70/40mm Hg.

Q2
SBA

A 29-year-old male presents with colicky abdominal pain, abdominal distension, vomiting and absolute constipation of 2 days' duration. He had undergone a laparotomy for a stab injury to his abdomen 1 year ago.

On examination, his temperature is 100°F and his pulse rate is 102/minute. The abdomen is distended with a well healed midline scar. The abdomen is generally tender but with no evidence of peritonitis or masses. The bowel sounds are hyperactive. No external herniae are identified.

His Hb is 14g/dL and WCC is 12,000/mm^3 (84% neutrophils and 10% lymphocytes).

What is the most likely clinical diagnosis in this patient?

a. Acute pancreatitis.
b. Acute cholecystitis.
c. Acute small bowel obstruction due to adhesions.
d. Acute diverticulitis.
e. Perforated appendicitis.

Q3
SBA

An 81-year-old male presents with abdominal colic, abdominal distension, vomiting and progressive constipation of 1 week's duration. During the last month he has been feeling generally unwell and increasingly tired. During the same period, he admits having a change in the pattern of his bowels towards constipation with bouts of liquid stools at times. He has had a cholecystectomy 20 years ago.

His primary care physician found him to be anaemic. His haemoglobin is 8.5g/dL

What is the diagnosis which needs to be excluded in this patient?

a. Diverticular disease.
b. Left colon cancer.
c. Chronic peptic ulcer disease.
d. Chronic pancreatitis.
e. Small bowel obstruction due to adhesions.

Q4
True/False

Factors which should be taken into consideration in making a diagnosis of the cause of acute intestinal obstruction are:

a. A past history of abdominal surgery.
b. The age of the patient.
c. A previous history suggestive of diverticular disease.
d. A previous history of surgery for bowel cancer.
e. That the patient is known to have gallbladder stones.

Q5
True/False

Acute intestinal obstruction due to adhesions:

a. Usually involves the small bowel.
b. Will respond to non-operative management.
c. Is complicated by bowel perforation.
d. Will lead to renal failure.
e. In the elderly, colon cancer should be excluded before establishing a diagnosis of adhesions as the cause of obstruction.

Q6
True/False

Causes of acute intestinal obstruction include:

a. Meconium ileus.
b. Diverticular disease.
c. Ulcerative colitis.
d. Intestinal atresia.
e. Meckel's diverticulum.

Q7
True/False

In patients with acute intestinal obstruction the following are true/false with regard to imaging:

a. Transverse bands which traverse across the bowel is characteristically seen in small bowel obstruction.
b. Small bowel is considered as pathologically dilated, if the maximum diameter is more than 5cm.
c. A dilated large bowel is seen mostly in the periphery of the film.
d. Caecal dilatation is considered significant when it is 10cm or more.
e. In the elderly with intestinal obstruction, contrast CT scans are associated with a risk of aspiration.

Q8
True/False

Which of the following features suggest impending ischaemia to a segment of bowel in patients with acute small bowel obstruction due to adhesions?

a. Colicky abdominal pain.
b. Deteriorating general condition.
c. Rise of pulse rate.
d. Localised abdominal tenderness.
e. A cough associated with a sharp increase in abdominal pain.

Answers overleaf

Self-assessment answers

Q1 1. (a), 2. (c), 3. (b), 4. (d).

Q2 (c).

Q3 (b).

Explanatory notes

In an elderly patient presenting with features of intestinal obstruction with a history of abdominal surgery, a diagnosis of adhesions should not be entertained until intra-abdominal malignancy is excluded.

Q4 a. (T), b. (T), c. (T), d. (T), e. (T).

Q5 a. (T), b. (T), c. (T), d. (T), e. (T).

Q6 a. (T), b. (T), C. (F), d. (T), e. (T).

Q7 a. (T), b. (T), c. (T), d. (T), e. (T).

Q8 a. (F), b. (T), c. (T), d. (T), e. (T).

Chapter 14

Acute abdomen

Learning objectives

- To learn the clinical presentation of a patient with peritonitis due to perforatec diverticulitis.
- To recollect the causes of an acute abdomen.
- To learn the management of a patient with suspected peritonitis.
- To learn the treatment of perforated diverticulitis.
- To learn the diagnostic pathway for postoperative pyrexia.
- To learn to identify high-risk patients for deep vein thrombosis (DVT) and prophylactic and therapeutic treatment for DVT.
- To learn the pathways for methicilin-resistant *Staphylococcus aureus* (MRSA) and *Clostridium difficile* infections in a secondary care setting.

Case scenario

A 77-year-old lady is found collapsed at home. She has had abdominal pain for 1 week and has been treated by her primary care physician for gastroenteritis. In the early hours of the morning she developed severe pain and was found collapsed in the toilet by her daughter who lives with her. During the last 2 months she has experienced intermittent abdominal colic, constipation and loose stools. She is awaiting an appointment from the hospital to see a surgeon. She has had a myocardial infarction 10 years previously. She is on aspirin and statins.

On examination, she is morbidly obese with a BMI of 44. She looks unwell and dehydratec. Her temperature is 38.8°C, pulse rate is 120/minute and RR is 22/minute. Her BP is 100/60mm Hg. The abdomen is distended and tender to palpation. The tenderness is most pronounced in the left lower quadrant. Both her femoral pulses are felt as well as her pedal pulses.

The results of the initial investigations are:

- White cell count 18,000/mm^3.
- Serum amylase 123U/L.
- Her abdominal X-ray has dilated small bowel and large bowel loops.
- An erect chest X-ray shows a rim of air under the diaphragm (Figure 1).

The most likely clinical diagnosis: peritonitis due to a perforated viscus.

She has perforated a gas-containing viscus in the peritoneal cavity. The severe pain she experienced in the early hours of the morning is compatible with this catastrophe.

The likely conditions compatible with this clinical picture include a perforated peptic ulcer in the stomach or duodenum, a perforated stomach cancer, appendicular or caecal perforation in the right colon and diverticular or tumour perforation in the sigmoid colon. Peptic ulcer, appendicular and diverticular perforations are the most common. Tumour perforations are rare.

A recent history of abdominal colic associated with altered bowel habits points to an obstructive lesion in the colon such as a diverticular mass/stricture or a cancer. Absence of a previous history of dyspepsia, loss of appetite and NSAID therapy makes peptic ulcer or perforated gastric cancer less likely. Therefore, the most likely condition is perforated sigmoid diverticulitis. This is also supported by the presence of severe tenderness in the left iliac fossa. The clinical picture of sepsis and dehydration is commonly seen in colon perforations because of the toxic effects of faecal peritonitis.

Acute appendicitis is uncommon in this age group. However, when it occurs, the clinical presentation may be atypical.

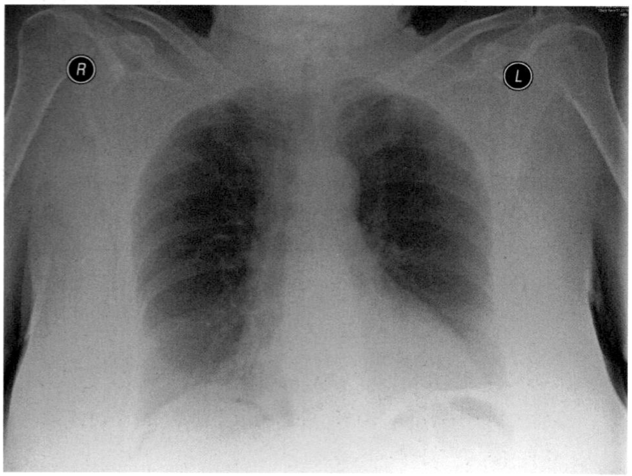

Figure 1. A chest X-ray showing a rim of air under the diaphragm.

In the elderly, perforated appendicitis presenting with a clinical picture of peritonitis may cause diagnostic difficulties.

A leaking abdominal aortic aneurysm is another important condition to exclude in the elderly with abdominal pain, hypotension and collapse. However, it is clear that this patient has perforated a gas-containing viscus because of the free abdominal gas.

Progress of the patient

- Intravenous fluids are commenced with Hartmann's solution.
- A haematological and renal liver profile, and electrolyte levels are requested.
- A catheter is inserted and hourly urine output recorded.
- A nasogastric tube is inserted.
- Blood cultures are obtained.
- A broad-spectrum antibiotic (e.g. cefuroxime or cefotaxime) together with metronidazole 500mg are administered intravenously.
- Two units of blood are cross-mached.
- An ECG +/- ECHO are performed.
- An urgent abdominal CT scan is arranged.
- Intermittent pneumatic calf compression is commenced for DVT prophylaxis.
- A CVP line is inserted.
- The abdominal and pelvic CT scan identify a mass lesion in the sigmoid colon with free intraperitoneal air and fluid in the peritoneal cavity suggestive of acute diverticular perforation. No air is seen in the bladder to suggest a vesicocolic fistula. The liver is normal. The large bowel is dilated up to the sigmoid colon. Generalised dilatation of the small bowel is noted.

Why is colonoscopy not considered in this patient?

A colonoscopy in the setting of acute diverticulitis will increase the risk of perforation.

The diagnosis of acute diverticulitis is made on clinical assessment. An ultrasound scan/CT scan is useful to assess mass lesions, the presence of fluid collections and the degree of bowel dilatation secondary to an obstructing lesion. Intraluminal assessment with colonoscopy or a barium enema is deferred because of the risk of perforation. In uncomplicated diverticulitis without evidence of suppuration, stricture formation or internal fistulae, the majority of patients will respond to antibiotics. A colonoscopy or barium enema is performed, once the acute episode is resolved, for assessment of the diverticular disease and also to exclude cancer.

Progress of the patient

- Serum Na 140mmol/L.
- Serum K 3.2mmol/L.
- CVP +2.
- Hourly urine output is 20ml/minute.
- The patient is hydrated. The perfusion rate is increased with CVP monitoring.
- Hourly urine output improves to 30ml and the serum K increases to 4.2mmol/l after IV potassium replacement.
- CVP +8.
- The patient receives intermittent pneumatic calf compression.
- Low-molecular-weight heparin is not given because the anaesthetist is planning to insert an epidural for postoperative pain relief and suggests deferring the heparin until the epidural is positioned.

Progress of the patient

- Informed consent is obtained explaining the:
  - benefits and risks of the procedure (a laparotomy and most likely a Hartmann's operation) highlighting the risk of infection, bleeding, DVT, pulmonary embolism and postoperative adhesions;
  - need to have a colostomy because the intended procedure is most likely to be a Hartmann's operation;
  - possibility of reversal;
  - possibility of a permanent colostomy;
  - possibility of discovering a cancer perforation.
- Her daughter who is the next of kin is informed and is involved in the decision making process as to the best option for the patient.
- The stoma nurse is introduced. The stoma nurse marks the sites of the stoma both on the left and right side, in the event that the patient may need an ileostomy.
- She undergoes an emergency laparotomy.
- A perforated inflammatory diverticular mass which is adherent to the bladder with fluid in the left iliac fossa and pelvis is seen. The colon is oedematous but viable and dilated up to the caecum. There are no diverticulae in the right colon. Free fluid in the peritoneal cavity is noted. Inventory of other intraperitoneal organs is normal.
- The surgeon decides to perform a Hartmann's procedure. The inflammatory mass in the sigmoid colon is resected. The distal stump of the sigmoid colon is divided using a stapling device. The distal site is marked with a non-absorbable suture for future identification of the stump. The descending colon is mobilised and a proximal end colostomy is formed in the left iliac fossa. The left ureter is identified carefully during the dissection. The peritoneum is washed with saline. A wide-bore non-suction drain is placed in the pelvis. Mass closure of the abdominal muscles is completed. Clips are used for skin closure.

Diverticulae are outpouchings of the colon. An important feature of diverticulae is that they do not contain all layers of the colonic wall. The most common site is the sigmoid colon. Asymptomatic diverticular disease is common in western societies.

The word diverticulitis refers to inflammation of the diverticulae caused by an obstruction to the neck of the diverticulum leading to stagnation and infection. Inflammation can lead to suppuration causing a diverticular abscess.

Perforation of the abscess will lead to a localised or generalised peritonitis. This may be purulent or faecal. Faecal peritonitis carries a very high mortality. If untreated, it leads to gram negative septicaemia, toxaemia and death.

An inflamed diverticular mass may become adherent to adjacent structures such as the bladder. It may perforate through the bladder wall causing a vesicocolic fistula. A vesicocolic fistula may present as an acute presentation when the abscess perforates into the bladder or sometimes as a chronic event when the fistulous tract is eventually formed due to recurrent episodes of inflammation of the diverticular mass adherent to the bladder. These patients may complain of pneumaturia, the passage of air when they pass urine.

Recurrent episodes of inflammation will lead to a diverticular stricture creating a picture of chronic large bowel obstruction which may be indistinguishable from a malignant stricture.

A chronic diverticular stricture may pose a diagnostic challenge even after a CT or barium enema, colonoscopy and at laparotomy. The final diagnosis may only be reached on histology following complete excision of the lesion.

What is a Hartmann's procedure?

A Hartmann's procedure is performed for lesions such as obstructing cancers or diverticulitis in the sigmoid colon when the operating surgeon decides against an anastomosis of the two ends of the divided colon after resecting the lesion. The decision on whether to perform an anastomosis or not is related to the perceived risk of a leak. An established infection in the peritoneal cavity, as in perforated diverticulitis, is often considered as a contraindication to primary anastomosis. The safest option is to close the distal end of the bowel leaving it as a 'stump' in the pelvis and to exteriorise the proximal end as an end colostomy in the left iliac fossa. If the distal stump is long enough, the distal limb may be brought out as another end colostomy. This is rarely possible in perforated diverticulitis. In cases of obstructed sigmoid cancer there may be sufficient length for the distal end to be exteriorised. The advantage of exteriorising the distal end is that it makes the reversal of the colostomy easier because both ends are easily recognisable. If the distal end is exteriorised it is called a distal mucous fistula. The decision is made depending on the length of the distal stump.

Progress of the patient

- Intravenous broad-spectrum antibiotics (e.g. cefuroxime or cefotaxime) and metronidazole 500mg t.d.s. are continued.
- Subcutaneous low-molecular-weight heparin and pneumatic calf compression are continued for DVT prophylaxis.
- This patient is obese, septic and is likely to be immobile postoperatively for a period of time. She is in the high-risk category for DVT.
- Chest physiotherapy is commenced and the patient is mobilised out of bed and encouraged to move. She refuses because with her weight and the laparotomy wound she simply finds it difficult to move around.
- Oral sips are commenced on the second postoperative day. The passage of flatus is observed on the third postoperative day. Oral intake is increased and a soft diet with high protein enteral feeding is commenced.

Progress of the patient

- The abdominal drain is removed on the fourth postoperative day.
- On the fifth postoperative day she complains of abdominal pain. She appears unwell. A temperature spike is noted in the temperature chart which was reported by the night staff and a septic screen has already been commenced by the night on-call officer.
- Bloods have been sent off for an FBC, CRP and blood culture. A sample of urine is sent for culture.
- She has a dry cough but is not producing sputum.
- She is already receiving chest physiotherapy.
- Her cannula site does not look infected or inflamed.
- Her CVP line has already been removed on the third postoperative day. There is no swelling in the neck.
- She has no leg or calf pain but both legs are slightly swollen.
- She does not look dyspnoeic but is clearly not cheerful.
- She has a chest X-ray which shows no evidence of pulmonary infection or effusion.
- Her WCC count has increased to 16,000mm^3 and her CRP is 125mg/dL. The WCC was 12,000mm^3 on the third postoperative day.
- The surgeon removes the abdominal dressings and inspects the wound. There is a swelling with overlying inflammation of the skin involving the lower half of the laparotomy wound which extends to the suprapubic region.

Progress of the patient

- The nurse is instructed to remove the lower five clips to open the swollen area. A collection of purulent fluid is released from the lower half of the wound. A sample is collected for culture. The wound is opened up in the lower half and irrigated with saline. The nurse is instructed to continue twice a day dressings as there is a significant collection and an obvious wound infection.
- There is no evidence of deep abdominal wall dehiscence.
- It is very likely that this may be the reason why she has felt unwell during the last 48 hours.

What is the next step?

- An urgent CT scan is requested to exclude an intra-abdominal collection.
- The antibiotic policy should be discussed with the consultant microbiologist. A Gram stain should be done straight away. If gram-positive cocci are seen, methicillin-resistant *Staphylococcus aureus* (MRSA) needs to be excluded. The laboratory should inform the surgical team immediately.

Progress of the patient

- The Gram stain shows gram-positive cocci.
- The microbiologist suggests adding a glycopeptide intravenously and not to discontinue the broad-spectrum antibiotic plus metronidazole regime until MRSA is confirmed.
- The patient is transferred to a cubicle for isolation as per the MRSA protocol of the hospital.

MRSA or methicillin-resistant *Staphylococcus aureus* is an organism that is resistant to commonly used antibiotics. Methicillin was an antibiotic used many years ago to treat patients with *Staphylococcus aureus* infections. Some individuals can become carriers of MRSA. MRSA organisms are often associated with patients in hospitals. The mere isolation of MRSA in a patient does not mean that they need treatment. Systemic antibiotics are indicated to treat MRSA infection only if there are clear clinical features of infection supported by blood test results.

If MRSA is isolated in a hospital-based patient it is important that strict measures are undertaken to prevent the spread of MRSA to other patients. The procedure is termed contact isolation.

Clinical points

- Principles of contact isolation:
  - the patient can be treated in the general surgical ward in a cubicle;
  - hand washing is a must, after touching either the patient or anything in contact with the patient;
  - the attending staff is advised to have short sleeves and to remove wrist watches;
  - the door should be kept closed;
  - patients can entertain visitors if they have no illness;
  - they can be discharged safely home once they become well;
  - when there are no signs of infection the antibiotics can be discontinued in consultation with the microbiologist.

The microbiologist is concerned because this patient is ill and although the broad-spectrum antibiotic covers *Staphylococcus aureus*, it does not cover MRSA. Therefore, if gram-positive cocci are seen and the patient is septic, it is advisable to add a glycopeptide to the antibiotics which she is already on as the treatment for MRSA. Once MRSA is isolated the other antibiotics may be discontinued. The microbiologist closely monitors the antibiotic policy with repeated swabs.

Progress of the patient

- The swabs are positive for MRSA.
- The microbiologist advises to stop the broad-spectrum antibiotic plus metronidazole and to continue with a glycopeptide.

Clinical points

- Antibiotic policy for MRSA infection:
  - systemic antibiotics are indicated to treat MRSA infection only if there are clear clinical features of infection supported by blood test results;
  - once the wound shows clear signs of healing and is no longer infected all antibiotics can be discontinued in consultation with the microbiologist;
  - if blood cultures are positive for MRSA, systemic antibiotics should be continued for a period of 14 days.

The main objective during the assessment of patients for postoperative pyrexia is to look for a cause. In an obese lady who has undergone major surgery for intra-abdominal sepsis, continuing infection is one of the commonest postoperative complications. A common site of sepsis is the wound.

It is not uncommon for obese patients to develop basal atelectasis because of breathing problems related to sedation and weight. However, pyrexia related to basal pulmonary atelectasis usually appears earlier than the fifth postoperative day.

If a patient develops high fever and chest signs during the first 24 hours of major surgery, aspiration pneumonitis should be suspected.

Line and catheter-related sepsis is high on the list by the fifth postoperative day. However, wound-related sepsis and intra-abdominal sepsis will be the most likely sites of infection in this obese patient who has undergone emergency surgery for intra-abdominal suppuration.

Deep venous thrombosis may occur with minimal physical signs in obese patients who are immobilised. This is another cause of postoperative pyrexia. This lady simply refuses to move postoperatively.

A useful mnemonic for recalling the causes of postoperative pyrexia is to remember the seven Cs:

- Chest.
- Cut (wound).
- Cannula.
- Catheter.
- Central line.
- Collection (of pus in the wound or intra-cavity).
- Calves (DVT).

The investigations requested and procedures carried out during a septic screening are shown in Table 1.

Table 1. Investigations requested and procedures carried out during a septic screening.

- FBC.
- Inflammatory marker levels: erythrocyte sedimentation rate (ESR), CRP.
- Chest X-ray.
- Urine examination.
- Line site cultures. The central line is removed and the tip is sent for culture. The peripheral cannulae are sited and a swab is taken if inflamed.
- Blood cultures.
- Wound site inspection. The clips or sutures are removed from the areas which appear to be under tension and inflamed to release the purulent material. The fluid is collected for culture or multiple swabs are taken.
- Abdominal CT/ultrasound scans.

Progress of the patient

- The patient's temperature settles with the release of pus from the wound.
- Her CT scan does not show any evidence of intra-abdominal collections. Wound discharge ceased rapidly and she is feeling better. She is keen to go home as she has good family support.
- The dietician is keeping her on high levels of enteral nutrition.
- On the 14th postoperative day, the tissue viability nurse inspects the wound. There is no oozing. The base of the wound appears red with new granulation tissue. There is no pus. The tissue viability nurse, in consultation with the ward sister and surgeon, decides that the wound can be managed on an outpatient basis by the wound care nurse.
- It is decided to continue subcutaneous low-molecular-weight heparin because the patient is still reluctant to walk with confidence. Her husband is keen to take her home as she has a better environment to walk around inside the house. The husband is retired and is available to help.
- She is on a normal diet now with protein supplements. She is gaining her appetite.
- The microbiologist approves the decision to discontinue all antibiotics because the wound is no longer infected and shows clear signs of healing. Her blood cultures have never been positive.
- She has now completed 7 days of glycopeptides. The intravenous antibiotics are discontinued prior to discharge home.

Progress of the patient

- The day before discharge, she complains of abdominal pain. She also informs the nurses that the contents in the bag are watery and very smelly. She is feeling unwell again. She has a pyrexia of 38.8°C. Her abdomen is slightly tender.
- The problem is discussed with the microbiologist.
- A stool sample is requested to test for a *Clostridium difficile* infection. The sample is collected in a leak-proof container and is despatched immediately.
- The surgeon requests an urgent repeat CT scan to exclude an intra-abdominal collection.
- The main concern is whether she is developing pseudomembranous colitis due to *Clostridium difficile* infection.
- The repeat CT scan shows no evidence of a new collection. There is some dilatation of the small and large bowel but no evidence of obstruction.

What is pseudomembranous colitis?

Pseudomembranous colitis is an infection of the colon caused by *Clostridium difficile* (*C. difficile*) which occurs in individuals who have previously been on antibiotic therapy.

C. difficile is one of the commonest hospital-acquired infections. Not infrequently, the non-infectious form of *C. difficile*, the 'spores', are found in hospital environments. The spores cannot cause infection directly but when ingested they transform into the active infectious form and cause serious infections.

The organism produces two toxins, toxins A and B, which cause damage to the wall of the bowel. Patients can become very septic and bowel perforations may occur.

The laboratories can check for the presence of *C. difficile* toxin, the results of which can be available in 2-3 hours.

Progress of the patient

- She is found positive for *C. difficile*.
- The microbiologist recommends metronidazole 400mg t.d.s. orally for 10 days.
- It is suggested that if no improvement is observed in 5-7 days, this can be changed to vancomycin 125mg t.d.s. orally for a period of 14 days.
- Her diarrhoea settles on the third day of therapy and she is feeling better.
- She is discharged home on the seventh day of treatment on oral metronidazole which she has tolerated well.
- Her husband is reassured that he has no major risk of acquiring this infection but is advised to use common sense in handling the bag contents.

Clinical points

- Antibiotic policy of *Clostridium difficile* infection:
  - in mild colitis, stopping the antibiotics that the patient is already on may be sufficient;
  - metronidazole or vancomycin are the two most commonly used antibiotics;
  - the duration of therapy is 10 days orally.

Progress of the patient

- Three days after discharge, she develops pain in the right leg and calls her primary care physician. On a home visit he observes that her right lower limb is swollen. He suspects deep vein thrombosis. She is admitted.
- An urgent duplex venous scan is arranged.
- An adherent clot is seen in the right femoral vein.
- The D-dimer assay is positive.

How useful is a D-dimer assay in the diagnosis of DVT?

Thrombus formation is normally followed by an immediate fibrinolytic response. The fibrinolytic response generates plasmin which causes the release of fibrin degeneration products which predominantly contain D-dimers. The absence of a rise of D-dimers implies that thrombosis may not have occurred.

High concentrations of D-dimers are not specific to making a positive diagnosis because of false positives which occur in other disorders such as malignancy, pregnancy and after operations. However, the lack of rising D-dimers has a high negative predictive value and is useful in excluding deep vein thrombosis in conjunction with clinical findings.

Progress of the patient

- Baseline bloods are sent off for analysis: FBC and platelet count, and a urea, electrolyte and liver profile.
- She is commenced on subcutaneous low-molecular-weight heparin.
- Warfarin therapy is commenced after the first dose of heparin.
- The INR is obtained daily until it is within range for 2 successive days. This is because the INR in the early stages of warfarin therapy is raised due to low levels of factor VII but full anticoagulation is not achieved until other vitamin K-dependent clotting factors (II, IX, X) become depleted. This usually takes about 3-5 days.

The standard initial management of deep vein thrombosis has traditionally been intravenous unfractionated heparin and maintenance therapy with warfarin. The low-molecular-weight heparins have now replaced unfractionated heparin. The main advantages are:

- Activated partial thromboplastin time (APTT) testing is not required.
- No infusion.
- Once daily dose.

The UK Haemostasis and Thrombosis Task Force guidelines on anticoagulation are shown in Table 2.

Table 2. Haemostasis and Thrombosis Task Force guidelines on anticoagulation.

- Patients should receive heparin for at least 4 days.
- Treatment of heparin is discontinued when the INR is within the therapeutic range for 2 consecutive days and warfarin is continued.
- A full blood count and platelet count are repeated after 5 days to look for heparin-related thrombocytopenia.
- A patient with a first episode of a proximal vein thrombosis should receive anticoagulants for 6 months, with a target INR of 2.5. The length of anticoagulation is under debate.
- A vena cava filter should be considered if anticoagulation is contraindicated.

This patient is not on any drug that interacts with her anticoagulant treatment. She is now off antibiotics.

Clinical points

- The drugs that interact with anticoagulants are:
  - macrolyte antibiotics (e.g. erythromycin);
  - non-steroidal anti-inflammatory drugs;
  - tamoxifen.

Mid Cheshire Hospitals NHS
NHS Foundation Trust

Patient identification

Contraindications to low-molecular-weight heparin (LMWH)

High risk of bleeding	Yes ☐	No ☐
On oral anticoagulants within therapeutic range	Yes ☐	No ☐
Raised INR	Yes ☐	No ☐
Creatinine clearance <30ml/min	Yes ☐	No ☐

Consider sucutaneous unfractionated heparin or reduced dose LMWH

Heparin-induced thrombocytopenia

Medical high-risk factors (1 or more = high)

Risk factor	Yes/No
History of recent travel 3 hrs-4 weeks before or after onset of symptoms	
Age >60	
Obese BMI >30 (BMI = weight kg/height m^2)	
Coexisting COPD, IHD, CCF or previous stroke	
Extensive varicose veins	
Previous DVT/PE	
Family history DVT/PE in 2 relatives (1 a 1st degree relative)	
Pregnant/puerperium	
HRT or oestrogen-containing pill	
Acute illness/coexisting sepsis Raised WCC, temp. >38°C, early warning score >4	
Inflammatory bowel disease	
Nephrotic syndrome	
Malignancy/cancer treatment	
Hypercoagulative state e.g. Protein C or S, ATIII deficiency, Factor V Leiden, lupus anticoagulant, thrombophilia, Behcet's disease, myeloproliferative diseases, paroxysmal nocturnal haemoglobinuria	
Immobility/paraplegia e.g. spends >90% of day in bed or chair	
Dehydration	
Indwelling femoral vein catheter, central venous catheter	

Surgical high-risk factors

Risk factor	Risk score	Comments
All surgery lasting <30 minutes	Low	
Thoracotomy or abdominal surgery involving a midline laparotomy	High	
Intraperitoneal laparoscopic surgery lasting >30 minutes	High	e.g. laparoscopic cholecystectomy
Total abdominal hysterectomy including laparoscopically-assisted	High	
Vascular surgery (not intra-abdominal)	High	e.g. carotid, peripheral limb surgery
Major joint replacement surgery	High	e.g. hip, knee, shoulder
Surgery for fractured neck of femur	High	Start on admission to hospital
Major trauma, e.g. bilateral lower limb or pelvic fractures	High	Start as soon as cardiovascular stability obtained and clotting is normal
All other surgery lasting >30 minutes	High	
Non-operative admission with immobility	High	e.g. spends >90% of day in bed or chair
Indwelling femoral vein catheter, central venous catheter	High	

Thromboprophylaxis regime

Low risk
1. Early ambulation
2. Apply graduated compression stockings or intermittent pneumatic therapy
3. Patient education leaflet

High risk
1. Enoxaparin 40mg once daily
2. Intermittent pneumatic therapy in theatre and/or during periods of immobility
3. Prompt and early mobilisation post-operatively or as mobility improves
4. Patient education leaflet

Anti-embolic stocking indicated	Thigh length ☐		Knee length ☐
LMWH indicated	Yes ☐	No ☐	Unsure ☐
Mechanical prophylaxis indicated	Yes ☐	No ☐	
Information leaflet gven to patient	Yes ☐	No ☐	Unsure ☐
Anticoagulation with LMWH indicated on discharge	Yes ☐	No ☐	
Duration of anticoagulation	2 weeks ☐		4 weeks ☐
Blood card given for platelet count 2 weeks after commencement of anticoagulation	Yes ☐	No ☐	

Date of assessment	
Assessor (please print)	
Designation (Sr, SN, Dr)	

Figure 1. A hybrid integrated VTE risk assessment tool. *Prepared by Dennis H Harthern, Dr MD Winson and Dr S Willmott with contributions from Drs. Zahid Saleem, Jahnavi Samanuru and Eleftheriadou Viktoria.*

Could her DVT have been predicted and prevented?

She is in the high-risk category on account of her weight, the severity of illness, dehydration, sepsis, major surgery, prolonged anaesthesia and postoperative immobility.

NICE guidelines on the treatment and prevention of DVT have categorised patients who are at risk of developing DVT and recommend using a care pathway. It is expected that such nationally agreed guidelines will be taken into account when NHS hospital trusts create their own care pathways for DVT.

Audit tools (audit protocol, methodology and instruments for measurement) are being created by some trusts to assess, improve and enhance their performance. An audit cycle is assessed on a fixed time frame to facilitate care pathways to enhance the quality of care.

Such an audit tool created by an individual trust is shown in Figure 1.

Progress of the patient

- The patient is discharged after 8 days with a stable INR of 2.5. The risks and benefits of warfarin therapy are discussed.
- Follow-up in the haematology and surgical clinics is arranged. She is coping well with her colostomy bag. She receives excellent support from the specialist colostomy nurse who visits her.

Progress of the patient

- She is reviewed at 8 weeks accompanied with her husband.
- The risks and benefits of the reversal of Hartmann's procedure are discussed. Having understood the precise nature of the procedure the patient is happy to live with the colostomy rather than undergo a further major operation with a high risk.

Reversal of Hartmann's procedure is a major surgical operation and is associated with substantial morbidity and mortality. Approximately 40% of patients who undergo Hartmann's procedure will not have a reversal. Reversal is a feasible operation for selected patients, but there is a high complication rate. Advanced age and comorbidity are the primary reasons for not undergoing a reversal.

Suggested reading

1. National Institute for Health and Clinical Excellence. Venous thrombo-embolism. Reducing the risk of venous thrombo-embolism (deep vein thrombosis and pulmonary embolism) in inpatients undergoing surgery. NICE guideline, 2007: 46.
2. Tovey C, Wyatt S. Diagnosis, investigation, and management of deep vein thrombosis. *BMJ* 2003: 326: 1180-4.
3. Autar R. The management of deep vein thrombosis: the Autar DVT risk assessment scale re-visited. *Journal of Orthopaedic Nursing* 2003; 7: 114-24.

Self-assessment

Q1
EMQ

a. Caecal cancer.
b. Resolving diverticulitis.
c. Ulcerative colitis.
d. Complicated diverticulitis.
e. Acute pancreatitis.
f. Leaking abdominal aortic aneurysm.

Select the most likely clinical diagnosis from the conditions mentioned above for the case scenarios described below.

1. A 77-year-old-lady presents with abdominal pain of 3 days' duration. On examination she has a temperature of 38.8°C, a pulse rate of 100/minute and a RR of 18/minute. Her BP is 90/60mm Hg. She has marked tenderness in the left iliac fossa. The WCC is 18,000/mm^3 and serum amylase is 123U/L.
2. A 78-year-old lady who presents with fever, abdominal pain and tenderness in the left iliac fossa of 3 days' duration has responded to an IV broad-spectrum antibiotic and metronidazole. She is apyrexial with no abdominal tenderness. An aortic aneurysm is excluded with an ultrasound scan.
3. A 77-year-old obese lady is admitted having been found collapsed in the toilet. She complains of severe abdominal pain. She looks clammy. During the period of resuscitation of 2 hours with 2L of Hartmann's solution, her BP reading in the emergency department reads as 70/50mm Hg, 100/60mm Hg and 90/70mm Hg. She is apyrexial. Her abdomen is slightly distended and tender.

Q2
EMQ

a. Ulcerative colitis.
b. Diverticular stricture.
c. Vesicocolic fistula.
d. Abdominal aortic aneurysm.
e. Caecal cancer.

Match the clinical feature given below with the most appropriate condition mentioned above.

1. Pneumaturia.
2. Fluctuating BP during resuscitation.
3. Blood and mucous diarrhoea.
4. Left-sided abdominal colic.
5. Fe deficiency anaemia.

Q3
SBA

On the sixth postoperative day after a Hartmann's procedure for perforated diverticulitis, a 79-year-old obese female complains of feeling unwell and a lower abdominal ache. She has had a temperature spike of 39°C the previous night. Inspection of the wound reveals an area of swelling and erythema of the skin involving the lower one quarter of the midline laparotomy incision. The skin appears to be under tension underneath the clips.

She is already on a broad-spectrum antibiotic and metronidazole.

What is the most appropriate next step in the management of this patient?

a. Release the lower few clips and collect a sample of fluid for gram stain and culture.
b. Obtain a swab for culture but do not remove the clips because of the risk of a burst abdomen.
c. Add gentamycin as an additional antibiotic.
d. Perform an emergency laparotomy to exclude intra-abdominal suppuration.
e. Request an ultrasound scan.

Q4
True/False

a. Perforated acute appendicitis is a common cause of an acute abdomen in the elderly.
b. Absence of pneumaturia in the history excludes the diagnosis of a vesicocolic fistula.
c. Glycopeptides are used in the treatment of methicillin-resistant *Staphylococcus aureus* (MRSA) infection.
d. Oral metronidazole therapy is used in the treatment of *Clostridium difficile* infection.
e. Aspiration pneumonitis should be suspected if a patient develops high fever and chest signs during the first 24 hours of surgery.

Q5
True/False

The patient-related risk factors of venous thrombo-embolism (VTE) include:

a. Pregnancy.
b. Antiphospholipid syndrome.
c. Obesity (BMI >30Kg/m^2).
d. Paraproteinaemia.
e. Extremes of age.

Answers overleaf

Self-assessment answers

Q1 1. (d), 2. (b), 3. (f).

Q2 1. (c), 2. (d), 3. (a), 4. (b), 5. (e).

Q3 (a).

Q4 a. (F), b. (F), c. (T), d. (T), e. (T).

Q5 a. (T), b. (T), c. (T), d. (T), e. (F).

Chapter 15

Inflammatory bowel disease

Learning objectives

- To learn the natural history and clinical presentation of ulcerative colitis (UC).
- To appreciate the differences between UC and Crohn's disease.
- To learn the complications of inflammatory bowel disease (IBD).
- To learn the surgical options for IBD.

Case scenario

A 50-year-old accountant with a history of longstanding ulcerative colitis (UC) of 15 years' duration presents with a 6-week history of bloody diarrhoea, urgency and frequency. He is on 40mg of prednisolone and 2g of aminosalicylates a day. He had a course of infliximab infusion 6 months ago but this had to be discontinued because the patient experienced side effects. Due to intermittent flare-ups of the disease he has not been in full employment during the last year. He is also troubled with arthritis which is attributed to UC. The last colonoscopy after inflixmab therapy indicates pancolitis.

At the onset of the disease 15 years ago, the initial and subsequent histology was indeterminate colitis (IC) and the possibility of Crohn's colitis had been raised.

The most likely clinical diagnosis: exacerbation of ulcerative colitis.

The term 'inflammatory bowel disease' (IBD) includes patients with chronic inflammation of the bowel. The two major forms of IBD are ulcerative colitis (UC) and Crohn's disease.

This patient has longstanding pancolitis. The word pancolitis refers to colitis involving the rectum and the entire colon.

Ulcerative colitis is a chronic inflammatory condition of unknown aetiology. The disease is limited to the mucosa of the colon. The inflammation commences in the rectum and extends to the proximal colon with occasional extension to the distal ileum. This is called 'backwash ileitis'.

Due to chronic inflammation, the colonic mucosa loses its ability to absorb water and also loses its normal mobility. This leads to watery diarrhoea, abdominal colic, an urge to defecate and tenesmus. Tenesmus is the painful urge to defecate and this is due to proctitis.

Extra-intestinal manifestations are often described with UC. These include arthritis, sclerosing cholangitis, erythema nodosum, ankylosing spondylitis and scleroderma.

Ulcerative colitis is considered as a pre-malignant condition. Patients with longstanding pancolitis have a significant risk of developing colon cancer. The mucosa of chronic UC may undergo dysplastic changes. Those with high-grade dysplasia have a high cancer risk.

Clinical points

- Both ulcerative colitis and Crohn's disease are considered as pre-malignant conditions.

What is indeterminate colitis?

Indeterminate colitis (IC) is the term used by pathologists when there is a difficulty in distinguishing between UC and Crohn's disease after histological examination of colonic biopsies or colectomy specimens.

UC and Crohn's disease are two distinct diseases. Both can present with diarrhoea, abdominal pain and weight loss. The management principles are different. Therefore, it is important to differentiate between the two. Table 1 highlights the key issues between the two diseases.

Table 1. The key issues between ulcerative colitis and Crohn's disease.

Ulcerative colitis	Crohn's disease
◆ Involves only the large bowel.	◆ Involves any part of the gastrointestinal tract from mouth to anus.
◆ Affects only the mucosa (a mucosal disease).	◆ Full thickness of the bowel is affected (a transmural disease).
◆ No submucosal granulomata on histology.	◆ Submucosal granulomata are characteristic.
◆ Almost always commences from the rectum and ascends upwards to involve the proximal colon, usually in continuity.	◆ Common sites are the ileum and right colon. A segmental disease. The bowel in between is normal producing the so called 'skip lesions'.
◆ Anal disease is rare.	◆ Recurrent anal abscesses and fistulae are seen especially in young patients with small bowel Crohn's.

Continued

Table 1. The key issues between ulcerative colitis and Crohn's disease *continued*.

Ulcerative colitis	Crohn's disease
◆ Clinical manifestations are related to chronic mucosal inflammation, sepsis, dysplasia and complications.	◆ Clinical manifestations are related to chronic mucosal inflammation, sepsis, dysplasia and complications.
◆ Fibrotic strictures are rare.	◆ Fibrotic strictures are common.
◆ Complications: toxic colitis, toxic megacolon, dysplasia and cancer.	◆ Complications: recurrent intestinal obstructions due to fibrotic or chronic inflammatory strictures, internal fistulae, complex peri-anal abscesses and fistulae, toxic megacolon, dysplasia and cancer (obstruction, fistulation, inflammation).
◆ Medical treatment: - nutritional; - anti-inflammatory drugs, e.g. amino-salicylates (oral, suppository); - steroids (oral, suppository, enema, IM, IV); - antibiotics, e.g. metronidazole, ciprofloxacin; - TNF inhibitors, e.g. infliximab; - immunosuppressives - e.g. azathioprine, cyclosporin.	◆ Medical treatment: - nutritional; - anti-inflammatory drugs; - steroids; - antibiotics, e.g. metronidazole, ciprofloxacin; - TNF inhibitors; - immunosuppressives, e.g. azathioprine, cyclosporin.
◆ Strong evidence supports that maintenance therapy significantly reduces the risk of relapse.	◆ The evidence to support maintenance therapy is less strong but many physicians prefer maintenance therapy.
◆ Surgery: - ileal pouch anal anastomosis (IPAA); - total colectomy and ileorectal anastomosis; - panproctocolectomy and permanent ileostomy.	◆ Surgery: - bowel resection including panproctocolectomy; - stricturoplasty; - abscess drainage; - fistula resection.
◆ Evidence of good quality of life with pouch surgery.	◆ Pouch construction is contraindicated.
◆ Short bowel syndrome does not occur.	◆ Repeated resections can result in short bowel syndrome.

Construction of an ileal pouch is contraindicated in Crohn's disease because the disease can occur in the small bowel used to construct the pouch. Removal of the pouch is a complex procedure.

In most patients with UC who have had an ileal pouch anal anastomosis (IPAA), the quality of life (QOL) is greatly improved.

An ileal pouch may develop a complication called pouchitis, which means inflammation in the mucosa of the pouch.

Progress of the patient

- Hb 10g/dL.
- S B12 - normal.
- S folate - normal.
- Liver and renal profile - normal.
- The colonoscopy shows up extensive changes of colitis extending all the way to the caecum. Multiple biopsies are performed from the right, transverse and left colon, and from the rectum to confirm the diagnosis of UC and also to look for dysplasia (Figure 1).
- Upper GI endoscopy - normal.
- Small bowel follow through - no small bowel disease.

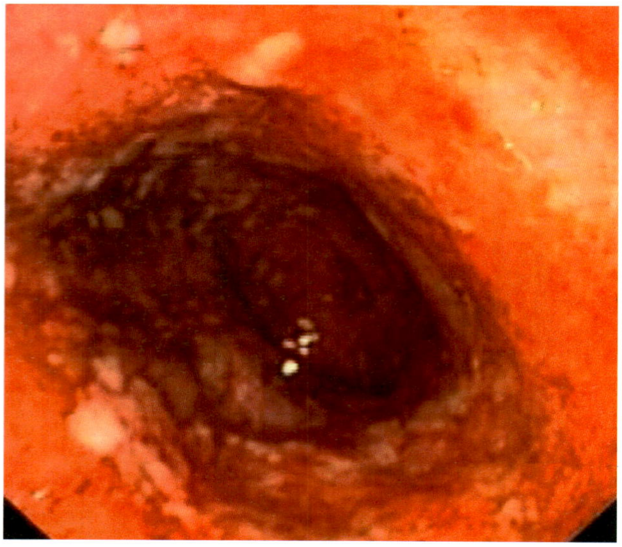

Figure 1. Colonoscopic appearance of ulcerative colitis. *Reproduced with permission from Hans Bjorknas, Gastrolab, Finland. www.gastrolab.net.*

Most patients with IBD can become anaemic due to chronic blood loss. Anaemia due to vitamin B12 deficiency may occur in patients with Crohn's disease affecting the ileum because the absorption of vitamin B12 occurs only through the terminal ileum.

A folate deficiency may also occur. The folate is largely absorbed in the jejunum. The deficiency will manifest in patients with short bowel syndrome after multiple bowel resections for stricturing or fistulating Crohn's disease.

An upper GI endoscopy and small bowel follow through was performed in this patient because of the initial diagnosis of indeterminate colitis to look for any evidence of Crohn's disease.

This patient has developed intractable disease despite medical therapy. He is requesting surgery.

What is the next step?

- The risks and benefits of the surgical options are discussed. Because of the initial doubt of the diagnosis between UC and Crohn's disease, the patient has second thoughts about an IPAA.
- He is informed that an alternative would be to do a two-stage procedure: a total colectomy and once the pathological diagnosis is confirmed and Crohn's disease is excluded, an ileal pouch could be constructed as the second stage.
- This would allow the pathologist to request another specialist second opinion on the resected specimen. He is informed that the evidence indicates a better quality of life with an IPAA.
- He is also informed of all the complications related to major surgery and a small risk of impotence and pouchitis.
- He is also informed that there is no guarantee that his arthritis will get better after surgery.

Progress of the patient

- After a period of deliberation the patient finally declines pouch surgery as he does not want to go through a two-stage procedure and certainly does not want to take a risk. His best friend has a bag and he has convinced him that it is not a problem.
- He opts for a pan-proctocolectomy and permanent ileostomy after being counselled by the medical gastroenterologist, stoma nurse and dietician.

What is pouchitis?

Pouchitis is a late sequel of IPAA surgery. This is a non-specific inflammatory condition of the ileal pouch which can mimic inflammatory bowel disease. It may occur as either a single attack or recur with intermittent acute attacks separated by times of normal pouch function. In a small number of patients, chronic pouchitis develops requiring constant maintenance therapy. Rarely, the pouch may have to be removed.

The indication for surgery in this patient is a disabling disease which has become refractory to medical therapy. It is affecting his lifestyle and employment. The other indications for surgery for inflammatory bowel disease are toxic megacolon, dysplasia (a risk for developing cancer) or cancer.

Individuals with longstanding UC and Crohn's disease are at an increased risk of developing colorectal cancer. The risk increases with more extensive colonic involvement and the longer duration of the disease.

There is evidence that patients with primary sclerosing cholangitis and UC have a higher risk of developing colorectal cancer and cholangiocarcinoma.

What is toxic colitis?

Toxic colitis is a dangerous complication of both ulcerative colitis and Crohn's disease. This occurs during an acute exacerbation. The bowel becomes dilated and ischaemic. The patients become septic and develop features of an acute abdomen.

An emergency colectomy can be life-saving.

Progress of the patient

- The patient has a pan-proctocolectomy and a permanent ileostomy.
- The initial high output from the ileostomy stoma is controlled with codeine.
- The stoma nurse is actively involved in the management and follow-up which includes home visits.
- At the second clinic visit it is noted that he has already gained weight, has accepted the ileostomy well and has already reported back to work.

Surgical resection of the diseased colon and rectum leads to resolution of all gastrointestinal symptoms. However, the benefits of surgery for extra-intestinal manifestations are not established.

Suggested reading

1. Cater MJ, Lobu AJ, Travis SPL. Guidelines for the management of inflammatory bowel disease in adults. *Gut* 2004; 53: 1-16.
2. Kozuch PL, Hanauer SB. Treatment of inflammatory bowel disease: a review of medical therapy. *World J Gastroenterol* 2008; 14(3): 354-77.

Self-assessment

Q1
EMQ

a. Involves any part of the GI tract from mouth to anus.
b. A mucosal disease.
c. Full thickness of the bowel is affected.
d. Submucosal granulomata are characteristic.
e. Skip lesions.
f. Multiple recurrent anorectal fistulae.
g. Fibrotic bowel strictures are not uncommon.
h. Ileal pouch construction can be performed.
i. Pouch construction is contraindicated.
j. Short bowel syndrome is a recognised complication.

Match the statements above with the most appropriate condition below.

1. Ulcerative colitis.
2. Crohn's disease.

Q2
SBA

A 70-year-old patient with known ulcerative colitis presents with a 2-week history of abdominal pain and a marked increase in the frequency of stools. He is on prednisolone and aminosalicylates. The primary care physician has increased his prednisolone to 30mg a day. During the last 48 hours, the severity of pain has increased but his bowel frequency has almost stopped.

On examination he looks unwell and his pulse rate is 120/minute with generalised abdominal tenderness. There are no other signs of peritonitis. His WCC is 20,000mm^3. There is no gas under the right hemi-diaphragm.

What is the most appropriate next investigation in the management of this patient?

a. Colonoscopy.
b. CT scan of the abdomen and pelvis.
c. Gastrograffin enema.
d. CT cologram.
e. Repeat chest X-ray.

Q3
SBA

A 34-year-old male with intermittent abdominal pain of 1-month duration is admitted as an emergency with increasing colic, abdominal distension and vomiting for the last 3 days. He has no past history of abdominal surgery or alteration of bowels. He has not passed flatus or faeces for the last 2 days.

What is the most likely site of his bowel obstruction?

a. Duodenum.
b. Small intestine.
c. Right colon.
d. Splenic flexure.
e. Rectosigmoid junction.

Q4
SBA

A 28-year-old Caucasian male presents with recurrent colicky abdominal pain of 1-month duration. He has lost 10Kg in weight. He is scared to eat because of colic.

What is the most likely clinical diagnosis?

a. Irritable bowel syndrome.
b. Peptic ulcer disease.
c. Diverticular stricture.
d. Crohn's disease.
e. Tuberculosis.

Q5
SBA

A 40-year-old female presents with a 4-week history of diarrhoea with blood and mucus, and mild intermittent abdominal pain. Her appetite is normal but she has lost 2-3Kg in weight during the same period. Her Hb is 11g/dL. Abdominal examination is unremarkable. Rigid sigmoidoscopy done in the outpatient clinic up to 12cm shows inflammation in the rectum.

What is the most appropriate next step in the management of this patient?

a. Flexible sigmoidoscopy and biopsy.
b. Proctoscopy, rectal biopsy and barium enema.
c. Colonoscopy and biopsies.
d. CT colography.
e. Contrast CT scan of the abdomen and pelvis.

Q6
True/False

In relation to the cause of obstruction in question 3 above, the differential diagnosis could include:

a. Crohn's disease.
b. Small bowel lymphoma.
c. Tuberculous stricture.
d. Ulcerative colitis.
e. Chronic appendicitis.

Answers overleaf

Self-assessment answers

Q1 1. (b), (h), 2. (a), (c), (d), (e), (f), (g), (i), (j).

Q2 (b).

Q3 (b).

Q4 (d).

Q5 (c).

Q6 a. (T), b. (T), c. (T), d. (F), e. (F).

Chapter 16

The critically injured patient

Learning objectives

- To learn the priorities in the initial management of the critically injured patient.
- To understand the basis of the Advanced Trauma Life Support® (ATLS®) approach.

Case scenario

A 42-year-old male is admitted to the accident and emergency department following a road crash. He has fallen asleep at the wheel and crashed his car into a tree. He is conscious, drowsy and agitated. He is pale.

His vital parameters are as follows: pulse rate is 120/minute, blood pressure is 90/60mmHg and RR is 34/minute.

His shirt is blood-stained. A deep laceration with some oozing of blood and bubbling of air is seen in the left anterior chest wall. He does not smell of alcohol.

The trauma team is ready in the department, as they have been informed of his arrival in advance.

What is the next step?

- The team leader commences the **primary survey**.
- He speaks to the patient and asks for his name. The patient replies with difficulty. The team leader opens the patient's mouth to assess for fluid, blood or foreign bodies with the sucker in his other hand. The oral cavity is normal.
- The airway nurse places a facemask and adjusts the oxygen flow to 10L/minute. She tags the pulse oximeter to his right index finger. It reads an arterial oxygen saturation of 84%.
- The team leader stabilises the neck by placing both hands on the patient's jaw while standing at the head end and the nurse positions a rigid cervical collar.
- The patient is dyspnoeic, tachypnoeic and tachycardic. He is agitated and drowsy. His oxygen saturation is low. The team leader comments that these features suggest significant arterial hypoxaemia and cerebral hypoxia. He consults with the anaesthetist and decides to intubate and ventilate the patient. The anaesthetist inserts an endotracheal tube and ventilates the patient.
- The nurse removes the patient's blood-stained shirt by cutting it with scissors and the team leader inspects the chest. He comments that the patient has a sucking chest wound on the left anterior chest wall and evidence of fractured ribs. He percusses and auscultates the chest. He identifies that the patient has a left-sided haemopneumothorax.
- He comments that the heart sounds are audible and the neck veins are not engorged.
- The team leader inserts a 28G intercostal drain in the 4th intercostal space of the left chest in the midaxillary line.
- He positions a gauze swab to close the sucking chest wound to stop air being sucked in.
- While this is being carried out, the 'circulation doctor' places two wide-bore cannulae (12F) into the veins in the antecubital fossae of both arms. He collects blood for cross-matching, an FBC, a renal and liver profile, and glucose and blood alcohol levels. He commences IL of N saline to each line. The drip rate is adjusted at a rate of 1L/hour. He requests 5 units of blood to be cross-matched urgently. He also requests 2 units of blood as soon as they are ready. He then examines the abdomen for free fluid and checks the stability of the pelvis to account for the patient's pallor. He finds that the abdomen is slightly distended but that there is no clinical evidence of free fluid or obvious instability of the pelvis.
- The team leader instructs the nurse to document the neurological status of the patient before the patient was ventilated. The nurse comments that the patient was not alert but that he responded to vocal commands during the initial assessment.
- The patient is exposed completely by cutting all his clothes in preparation for the secondary survey.
- The team leader examines the genitals before catheterisation. No swelling, bruising or discolouration are noted in the scrotum. He then inspects the external meatus for blood. He inserts a 14F Foley catheter and instructs the nurse to measure urine volume in the bladder and to maintain an hourly output chart.

Progress of the patient

- The vital parameters now are a pulse rate of 112/minute and a BP of 100/60mm Hg.
- The patient is ventilated.
- The patient still looks pale.
- The team leader commences the **secondary survey**.
- The team leader conducts a thorough head to toe examination, commencing from the scalp. He looks for swelling, bruising, deformity and cracks by carefully feeling the scalp with both hands.
- With the assistant helping to release the cervical collar, he re-examines the neck for evidence of soft tissue and bony injuries.
- He then examines the chest systematically, inspecting the chest wall for further evidence of soft tissue and bony injuries, palpating to confirm rib fractures and surgical crepitus, which means the presence of air in the chest wall. He confirms the left-sided pneumothorax and re-assesses the heart sounds for any crackling noises which might indicate the presence of blood in the pericardium.
- The intercostal tube is swinging and the air entry to the right chest is satisfactory.
- He re-examines the abdomen. There is some bruising over the left hypochondrium and a swelling over the left lower chest wall in addition to the deformity of the left lower chest wall which he detected during the primary survey. He comments that the patient may have a splenic injury. He re-examines the pelvis for abnormal mobility and checks the long bones for soft tissue injury and fractures but does not find any abnormality.
- He instructs the team to 'log roll' the patient and examines the back of the neck, chest and abdomen.
- Whilst the patient is stabilised in the log roll position, he inserts his gloved finger into the rectum and comments that the level of the prostate is normal and that there is no blood on the examination finger.
- Whilst the second unit of blood is being transfused, he requests a focused assessment sonography for trauma (FAST) ultrasound.
- The team leader reassesses the vital parameters. The BP is still 100/60mm Hg despite a transfusion of 2 units of blood. The pulse rate is 112/minute and the pulse volume is still low.
- At the completion of the second unit of blood and while the infusion is being changed, the blood pressure suddenly falls to 95/60mm Hg. The rate of saline infusion is increased.
- The team leader decides that the patient needs a laparotomy because the patient is showing signs of haemodynamic instability.
- The FAST ultrasound reveals that this patient has free fluid in the peritoneal cavity with a swelling around the spleen. No fluid is identified in the pericardium.
- A chest and pelvic X-ray are taken without delay. The anaesthetist comments that there are fractures of the 5th to 8th ribs on the left side with a haemopneumothorax, that the position of the intercostal tube is satisfactory and that there is a faint soft tissue shadow in the right lung which is compatible with a pulmonary contusion.
- No pelvic fractures are seen on the X-ray.
- A lateral cervical spine X-ray is not performed because of the time constraints and the patient already has a cervical collar in position.

Progress of the patient

- The team leader summarises the patient's condition to the team: the patient has a Class III haemorrhage due to a haemothorax, multiple rib fractures on the left side, a contusional lung injury on the right side and intra-abdominal bleeding with haemodynamic instability.
- He instructs the team to wheel the patient to the operating theatre.
- He decides against an emergency CT to gain further information because the patient is becoming haemodynamically unstable.
- He calls the relatives and explains to them the injuries and the status of the patient. He informs them that the patient's condition is serious and that he needs an urgent exploration of his abdomen and a possible splenectomy. He also enquires from the relatives whether the patient has any allergies, is on any medications, has any past illnesses, and what time he may have consumed his last meal and drinks. He also informs the relatives on the information he obtained from the ambulance crew, that the vehicle had toppled over and that he was found crushed under the vehicle. The patient's wife tells him that prior to the incident, her husband had been at a party and he is likely to have a full stomach. He is not on any drugs and he has no allergies. He is vaccinated against tetanus.
- The patient is given a broad-spectrum antibiotic (e.g. cefuroxime 1.5g IV or gentamycin 80mg IV) and metronidazole 500mg IV.
- Laparotomy reveals 3L of blood in the peritoneal cavity, a deep laceration over the spleen with a haematoma, a contusion of the small bowel and a haematoma in the small bowel mesentery. The large and small bowel look viable. The rest of the intraperitoneal organs are normal.
- The surgeon performs a splenectomy. The anaesthetist decides to continue ventilation after surgery because of the severity of the bilateral chest trauma.
- The patient is taken to the ICU.
- The surgeon speaks to the relatives and explains the exact situation. He comments that the patient's condition is now critical but stable, and that the bleeding is under control.

What is a trauma team?

A trauma team consists of a team leader who is the most senior or experienced clinician, an airway doctor who is an anaesthetist and a circulation doctor. The airway doctor is assisted by the airway nurse and the circulation doctor is assisted by the circulation nurse. The team leader is assisted by a nurse who will also maintain the documentation. She will also liaise with the relatives.

This is the so called 'horizontal approach' to the management of the critically injured.

In reality, this ideal situation is not possible in most trauma facilities due to many constraints. However, in dedicated trauma centres in some parts of the world, this concept has now become routine practice.

Sometimes, only one clinician may be available to handle such emergencies. He is usually assisted by one nurse. This is the 'vertical approach'. That is, during the primary survey, he will attend to the airway, breathing and circulation in that order. This of course, is less satisfactory and may have an effect on the outcome.

What is the Advanced Trauma Life Support® (ATLS®) system?

The Advanced Trauma Life Support® course of the American College of Surgeons is a unique approach designed to optimise the initial management of critically injured patients.

Pioneering work by Donald Truncky and others has shown that critically injured patients die not only due to the severity of the injuries, but because of the inadequate care they receive, especially during the first hour. This is called the 'golden hour' following trauma.

Studies have shown that those patients who receive proper treatment during the first hour will have a much better chance of survival. Hypoxia and hypovolaemia are recognised as the two main causes of death during the first hour. Prompt recognition and vigorous treatment of hypoxia and hypovolaemia is shown to reduce mortality following trauma. The ATLS approach to trauma care is designed to address these issues.

What then is the difference between the conventional approach to the surgical management of a patient and the ATLS approach?

The conventional approach to the surgical management of a patient is to obtain a history, carry out a comprehensive clinical examination and to arrive at a differential diagnosis. The clinician will then arrange a set of investigations and formulate a plan of treatment. Studies have shown that this approach does not produce the desired outcome in the critically injured. The outcome depends on the prompt recognition and treatment of hypoxia and hypovolaemia and this will reduce deaths during the second peak of the trimodal distribution of trauma deaths. In the ATLS method, a regimented approach referred to as the primary and secondary survey is taught to achieve this objective.

What is meant by the trimodal pattern of trauma deaths?

In 1983, Truncky in his pioneering study identified that deaths after trauma follow a trimodal distribution. The first and largest peak of deaths, comprising 50% of the total, is seen immediately or within seconds of the injury. The second peak, 30% of deaths, occurs up to 4 hours later, while the third comprises those 20% of patients who die after 4 hours.

Those who belong to the first peak usually die from unsalvageable head injuries or major thoracic or abdominal vascular disruptions. Therefore, the only method of reducing the number of deaths in this group is to enhance preventive programmes such as seat belt legislation, strict enforcement of helmet use and drink driving laws.

In the ATLS teaching, the main emphasis is placed on the second peak. This is because the cause of death in the second peak is hypoxia and/or hypovolaemia that can be effectively treated to change the outcome. Many believe that appropriate intervention for patients in this group at the pre-hospital level (at the scene) or at the time of admission to the hospital offers the greatest potential in preventing unnecessary deaths. As a result, the provision and nature of pre-hospital and hospital trauma services have been profoundly affected all over the world. In particular, ambulance services, paramedic training and the concept of trauma centres have received considerable attention.

The third peak consists of all those who die after 4 hours. Many survive for days or weeks. These include patients who die due to multiple organ failure as a result of overwhelming sepsis. The deaths in this peak have fallen because of better intensive care facilities.

As shown in the case scenario the primary survey is ideally carried out by a team of doctors. The essential differences between the primary survey and the conventional approach are that:

- The initial assessment and treatment (resuscitation) will begin simultaneously.
- It attempts to recognise and treat the most likely immediate cause of death first.

What is meant by the 'most likely immediate cause of death'?

It is interesting to note that trauma kills people according to a pre-formed sequence!

Acute airway obstruction (A - AIRWAY) is the quickest killer of the injured. In fact, acute complete airway obstruction will kill a person in 3 minutes.

Inadequate breathing (B - BREATHING) is the second quickest killer of the injured. Inadequate breathing may be due to blunt or penetrating injuries to the chest.

A tension pneumothorax, massive haemothorax, flail chest and cardic tamponade are immediate life-threatening chest injuries.

Hypovolaemia (C - CIRCULATION) is the third quickest killer.

An external haemorrhage is easy to identify and is therefore easy to assess the severity. But it is often not easy to assess the severity of a concealed or hidden haemorrhage. Patients can bleed into five sites in the human body; the spaces where blood can collect. These five sites are the chest cavity, the peritoneal cavity, the pelvis, the retroperitoneal space and the thighs due to long bone fractures, especially in children. Of course, the peritoneal cavity, retroperitoneum and pelvis are interconnected but the main loss may be into one of these spaces.

Expanding intracranial haematoma (D - neurological DISABILITY) is the fourth killer. Therefore, during the primary survey, a quick assessment of the level of consciousness is made by the AVPU method.

- A - alert.
- V - responds to vocal stimuli.
- P - responds only to painful stimuli.
- U - unresponsiveness.

The Glasgow Coma Score (GCS) is calculated during the secondary survey (refer to Chapter 17).

(E) - is the Exposure. The patient must be completely stripped of all his clothes by cutting them off. Clothes should never be pulled off as they may aggravate an unstable spinal injury.

(F) - is the placement of a Foley catheter. As highlighted in the case scenario, the patient should not be catheterised if there is blood at the tip of the penis, or swelling or bruising of the scrotum, which may mean partial or complete rupture of the urethra. If there is any doubt this must be investigated further. If the bladder becomes distended during fluid resuscitation a suprapubic catheter may be inserted. One needs to be extra cautious if there is a pelvic fracture.

Secondary survey

The secondary survey will begin when the primary survey is completed, resuscitation is in progress and all vital signs are re-documented. However, if the vital signs show deterioration, it is most important to revert back to the primary survey again to identify and deal with the most life-threatening problem.

Clinical points

- If the vital signs show deterioration, it is most important to revert back to the primary survey again.

The main objective of the secondary survey is to perform a comprehensive assessment of the patient from head to toe in a systematic manner, as highlighted in the case scenario. This helps clinicians to arrive at a diagnosis with regard to the organ system/systems involved and to appreciate the severity of the condition.

As far as hypovolaemia is concerned, at the end of the secondary survey three types of patients are recognised:

- Patients who are haemodynamically normal.
- Patients who are haemodynamically stable.
- Patients who are haemodynamically unstable.

A patient is considered haemodynamically normal if the vital signs remain normal, once the resuscitation is reduced or discontinued. Haemodynamically stable patients are those who show signs of instability when the resuscitation is reduced. Haemodynamically unstable patients do not respond to resuscitation. They usually have catastrophic haemorrhage and emergency exploration of the affected region is mandatory as a life-saving measure.

Depending on the response to fluid resuscitation, at this stage the clinician will have arrived at a judgement as to the best course of action, as shown in the case scenario.

The history is important but should be left to the end of the secondary survey to save time for resuscitation. The mnemonic, AMPLE, is useful as it is easy to remember as an apple, although it is spelt as ample.

- A - allergies.
- M - medications.
- P - past illnesses.
- L - last meal.
- E - events related to the injury.

X-rays are not mandatory. The three X-rays which will assist the immediate management of the critically injured are:

- X-ray chest.
- X-ray pelvis.
- Lateral cervical spine.

Focused assessment sonography for trauma (FAST) ultrasound is available in many trauma facilities. The main objective is to recognise the presence of fluid in the peritoneum and fluid in the pericardium. A negative FAST ultrasound does not exclude concealed intra-abdominal bleeding.

Diagnostic peritoneal lavage (DPL) may be useful at times when a FAST ultrasound is not available. DPL is rarely used in the UK.

CT scans are useful to gain more objective information. However, their use is limited only to some patients who are haemodynamically stable.

It is most important to understand the major human factor during the management of the critically injured. The majority of critically injured patients arrive at unsocial hours and most are young males. The relatives must be spoken to by a senior responsible clinician and must be continually informed of the progress of the patient.

Progress of the patient

- The postoperative period is uneventful.
- The patient is given pneumococcal vaccination prior to discharge.
- Oral penicillin 250mg b.d. is commenced. He is advised to continue this dose indefinitely.
- He is advised to seek medical advice immediately if he develops infective symptoms such as pyrexia, malaise, shivering, etc., and the need to commence a full therapeutic dose of antibiotics.
- He is advised to keep a reserve supply of antibiotics at home and when on holiday.

What are the risks of infection post-splenectomy?

Overwhelming and sometimes fatal infections represent a life-long risk after surgical removal of the spleen. Encapsulated organisms are frequently involved in sepsis in patients who have undergone splenectomy. The risk is greater in the early months and years following splenectomy but persists throughout life. The risk of sepsis is higher in children. *Streptococcus pneumoniae* is the commonest cause of sepsis.

The British Committee for Standards in Haematology produced an update in 2002. The key points are:

- All splenectomised patients should receive pneumococcal immunisation.
- Patients not previously immunised should receive a *Haemophilus influenzae* Type B vaccine and meningococcal Group C conjugate vaccine.
- Influenza immunisation should be given.
- Life-long prophylactic antibiotics are still recommended (oral phenoxymethylpenicillin or erythromycin).
- Revaccination 5 years later is recommended.

Suggested reading

1. Truncky DD. Trauma. *Scientific American* 1983; 249(2): 20-7.
2. Royal College of Surgeons of England. Report of the Working Party on the Management of Patients with Major Injuries. London: Royal College of Surgeons of England, 1988.
3. Wyatt J, *et al.* The time of death after trauma. *BMJ* 1995; 310: 1502.
4. Davis JM, *et al.* Update of guidelines for the prevention and treatment of infection in patients with an absent or dysfunctional spleen. The British Committee for Standards in Haematology, 2002; http://www.bcshguidelines.com/pdf/SPLEEN21.pdf.

Self-assessment

Q1
EMQ

a. Cardiac tamponade.
b. Tension pneumothorax.
c. Multiple rib fractures.
d. Massive haemothorax.
e. Acute airway obstruction.
f. Bronchopleural fistula.
g. Open pneumothorax.

Select the most likely clinical diagnosis mentioned above for the case scenarios described below.

1. A 45-year-old male is admitted following a road crash. He is acutely dyspnoeic and has a stridor.
2. A 25-year-old male complains of left-sided chest pain following a fall. He has bruising on the posterior chest wall and normal air entry bilaterally. He is haemodynamically normal.
3. An 18-year-old male is seen shortly after a stab injury to his left chest. He is pale and hypotensive. Air entry is normal bilaterally. His neck veins are engorged.
4. A 22-year-old male is admitted after a fight. He complains of chest pain. He is dyspnoeic, pale and hypotensive. His neck veins are engorged.
5. A 33-year-old male is admitted after a fight. He complains of chest pain. He is dyspnoeic, pale, tachycardic and hypotensive.
6. On the 4th day after inserting a chest drain for a pneumothorax following a stab injury to the chest, the lung remains collapsed and a continuous bubbling of air is observed in the bottle.

Q2
EMQ

a. Haemothorax.
b. Tension pneumothorax.
c. Cardiac tamponade.
d. Pneumothorax.
e. Bronchopleural fistula.
f. Empyema.
g. Multiple rib fractures.
h. Pulmonary contusion.

Match the clinical feature given below to the most appropriate condition given above. Each option can be selected only once.

1. Hypotension.
2. Chest wound with bubbling of air.
3. Engorged neck veins.
4. Marked swelling of the face and neck.
5. Continuous bubbling of air in the intercostal drain bottle.

Q3 SBA

A 28-year-old man is admitted to the hospital following a road accident. The medical officer observes that the patient is dyspnoeic and pale and has a deep laceration in his right thigh.

What is the next step?

a. To speak to the patient.
b. To suture the right thigh wound.
c. To commence a saline drip.
d. To call a senior doctor.
e. To arrange for a chest X-ray.

Q4 True/False

The immediate life-threatening injuries following major trauma include:

a. Tension pneumothorax.
b. Massive haemothorax.
c. Multiple rib fractures.
d. Cardiac tamponade.
e. Open pneumothorax.

Answers overleaf

Self-assessment answers

Q1 1. (e), 2. (c), 3. (a), 4. (b), 5. (d), 6. (f).

Q2 1. (a), 2. (d), 3. (c), 4. (b), 5. (e).

Q3 (a).

Q4 a. (T), b. (T), c. (F), d. (T), e. (F).

Chapter 17

Head injury

Learning objectives

- To learn the significance of and be able to calculate the Glasgow Coma Score (GCS).
- To recollect the anatomy and pathophysiology of head injury.
- To learn the causes of secondary head injury and preventive measures.
- To learn the initial management of acute intracranial mass lesions.

Case scenario

A 21-year-old student is admitted with a history of assault following an argument in a pub. He was struck with a beer bottle on the right side of his head. His friend noted that he fell 'unconscious' immediately after the assault. The friend attempted to rouse him but he did not regain consciousness for about 15 minutes.

During the primary survey, his airway is normal, RR is 26/minute and pulse rate is 78/minute. BP is 130/80mm Hg.

The patient does not open his eyes to command but opens his eyes in response to painful stimuli. He withdraws from painful stimuli. His only verbal responses are incomprehensible sounds. The pulse oximeter reads an arterial oxygen saturation of 88%.

He has a 3cm laceration with surrounding contusion over the right temple. The right pupil is dilated to 6mm and there is a sluggish reaction to light. The left pupil is normal in size and reacts normally to light.

No blood is noted behind the ear drums, in the external ear or in the nasal passage.

The remaining examination including the thorax, abdomen, pelvis, spine and long bones is normal.

The most likely clinical diagnosis: a severe closed head injury with a possible mass effect.

This patient has a Glasgow Coma Score (GCS) of 8 and a dilated right pupil. He has a severe closed head injury. The dilated right pupil indicates a possible mass effect. His arterial oxygen saturation is 88%.

What is the next step?

- A primary survey is performed during which the patient is immediately intubated and ventilated (refer to Chapter 16).
- A secondary survey is performed.
- An urgent CT scan is arranged to assess the nature of the head injury.
- An intravenous infusion of N saline is commenced and blood pressure is closely monitored.

What is the Glasgow Coma Score (GCS)?

The Glasgow Coma Scale or Score (GCS)(Table 1) is the most widely used scoring system to quantify the level of consciousness following a traumatic brain injury. It is popular because it is a simple system and correlates well with the outcome following severe brain injury.

The system determines the best eye opening response, the best verbal response, and the best motor response in a numeric score as shown below. The score represents the sum of the scores of each category.

A score of 13 or higher correlates with a mild brain injury. A score between 9 to 12 is a moderate injury and 8 or less is a severe brain injury. Patients with a GCS of 8 or below are unconscious. The minimum score that can be obtained is 3.

Certain factors such as hypoxia, hypotension, narcotic drugs, alcohol intoxication, and metabolic disturbances may alter the GCS independently of the brain injury. Therefore, these factors may alter the level of consciousness.

A spinal cord injury will make the motor scale invalid. In severe orbital trauma, eye opening is impossible to assess.

Clinical points

- With a score at 8 or below the patient is unconscious.
- A score of 8 or below may be considered for intubation and ventilation because the airway is considered as unsafe.
- Factors other than the brain injury can make the patient unconscious.
- A concomitant spinal injury makes the motor scale invalid.

Table 1. Glasgow Coma Scale.

Eye opening	Verbal response	Motor response
Spontaneous = 4.	Normal conversation = 5.	Obeys commands = 6.
To voice = 3.	Confused = 4.	Localises = 5.
To pain = 2.	Inappropriate = 3.	Withdraws from pain = 4.
None = 1.	Incomprehensible = 2.	Flexion response (decorticate posture) = 3.
	No response = 1.	Extension response (decerebrate posture) = 2.
		No response = 1.

The Glasgow Coma Score of 8 indicates that this patient has received a severe head injury and he is unconscious. However, the precise nature of the brain injury cannot be ascertained by these physical signs or by the Glasgow Coma Score.

This patient may be developing, or has already developed, an extradural, subdural or intraparenchymal haematoma, subarachnoid haemorrhage, a diffuse axonal injury or a combination of these injuries.

He is brought in immediately after the injury. Therefore, the present clinical picture is most likely due to the injury to the brain as a direct consequence of the impact. This is referred to as a primary head injury.

What is a primary head injury?

A primary head injury is injury to the brain due to the impact at the time of the event. There is no treatment for the injury due to the initial impact. Therefore, the precise nature of the injury is less important in the initial treatment of this patient but it is important for definitive treatment.

What is more important is to prevent secondary brain injury. The initial treatment is focused on achieving this objective.

What is a secondary head injury?

A secondary head injury is the injury that occurs after the initial impact to an already injured brain. This may be caused by three factors. These are:

- Hypoxia.
- Hypotension.
- Increased intracranial pressure (ICP).

Structural changes from head injury may be gross or microscopic, depending on the mechanism and forces involved. Patients with less severe injuries may have no gross structural damage. Clinical manifestations vary markedly in severity and consequences. Injuries are commonly categorised as open or closed.

The main pathophysiological pathway of a brain injury is centred on ischaemic damage to the injured brain tissue. The lack of glucose and oxygen depletes cellular energy required to maintain electrical potentials and an ion gradient. Early ischaemia has been found to correlate with poor outcome and early mortality.

Primary brain injury stimulates the cells of the central nervous system (CNS) to produce a variety of mediators such as tumour necrosis factor and interleukin-6 that mediate toxicity.

Many of the clinical signs which are seen after an acute brain injury (pyrexia, neutrophilia and cerebral oedema secondary to disruption of the blood brain barrier) are believed to be caused by cytokine activity.

An injured brain is more susceptible to hypoxia, hypotension and increased ICP than a normal brain. Therefore, prevention of hypoxia is essential. In the presence of any evidence of impending or early hypoxia, immediate endotracheal intubation and ventilation is the most vital component in the initial management of patients with severe head trauma. This is why this patient is immediately intubated and ventilated. His oxygen saturation on admission was 88%.

Hypotension alone doubles the mortality risk compared with that of normotensive patients with severe head trauma. This is the reason why the patient is given an urgent intravenous infusion and his blood pressure is closely monitored.

NICE guidelines recommend maintaining arterial oxygen saturation above 90% and systolic blood pressure above 90mm Hg.

How does raised intracranial pressure cause secondary head injury?

The cranial vault is essentially a closed fixed bony box. Its volume is constant. This volume is described by the Monro-Kellie doctrine.

In 1783, Alexander Monro, a Scottish physiologist, deduced that the cranium was a rigid box filled with a nearly incompressible brain. Its total volume tends to remain constant. Any increase in the volume of cranial contents (e.g. brain, blood or cerebrospinal fluid [CSF]) will elevate intracranial pressure. Furthermore, if one of these three elements increases in volume, it must occur at the expense of the volume of the other two elements. In 1824, George Kellie confirmed many of Monro's early observations:

Intracranial volume (constant) =
brain volume + CSF volume + volume of the
mass lesion (haematoma)

Because the fluid is non-compressible, once the cranial vault is filled with blood or fluid, the pressure within the cranial vault will rise. This rise of intracranial pressure leads to interruption of cerebral blood flow by reducing the cerebral perfusion pressure. When an intracranial mass lesion or oedematous brain expands, initially the CSF and blood move into the spinal canal and extracranial vasculature, respectively. But beyond this further compensation is not possible and the ICP rises dramatically (Figure 1).

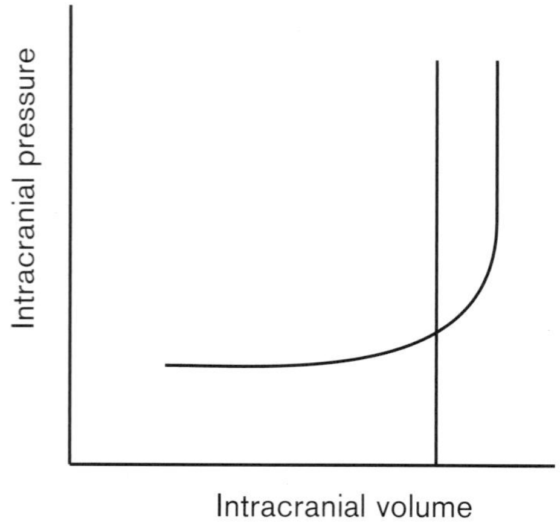

Figure 1. A graph demonstrating the relationship between intracranial pressure and volume.

An increased ICP leads to interruption of the cerebral blood flow by reducing the cerebral perfusion pressure.

Increased ICP is either due to a collection of blood in the extradural, subdural, subarachnoid, intraventricular spaces or in the brain parenchyma. This increase in pressure may also be due to oedema of the brain. The more damage the brain receives, the more it swells. This is termed cerebral oedema. In a hypotensive patient, even a small increase in ICP can be harmful.

A normal ICP is 5-15mmHg. Levels above 20mmHg are usually treated.

There is evidence that ICP monitoring reduces the mortality of patients with severe head injuries and is recommended for patients with severe head injuries. ICP monitoring is now a central part of critical care management for the severely brain-injured patient.

How significant is the finding of a dilated pupil with a sluggish light response in this patient?

The presence of a dilated pupil on the right side in this patient suggests a mass effect with increased intracranial pressure.

This is a very significant finding because it is an early sign of temporal lobe herniation. The occulomotor nerve (3rd nerve) becomes compressed between the free edge of the tentorium and the herniating temporal lobe. The pupillary abnormality initially occurs on the same side of the intracranial lesion.

Clinical points

- There is no treatment for the injury due to the initial impact and, therefore, the precise nature of the injury is less important in the initial treatment.
- Prevention of secondary brain injury by optimising oxygenation, ventilation and brain perfusion by avoiding hypoxia and hypotension is the key to immediate management.
- The Glasgow Coma Score on admission and the subsequent changes of the score is an important indicator of the response to therapy.
- The side on which the dilated pupil is located indicates the side of the intracranial mass lesion.
- Intracranial pressure monitoring is shown to improve the outcome of patients with severe head injuries.

Progress of the patient

- An emergency CT scan is performed. This reveals a right-sided extradural haematoma (Figure 2).
- The patient is transferred to the regional neurosurgical unit for an emergency craniotomy and evacuation of the haematoma.
- Blood pressure is 120/70mm Hg and arterial oxygen saturation is 96%.
- The regional neurosurgical unit advises administration of an intravenous bolus of mannitol (1g/Kg) and hyperventilation to maintain PCO_2 at 25-30mm Hg during the transfer.

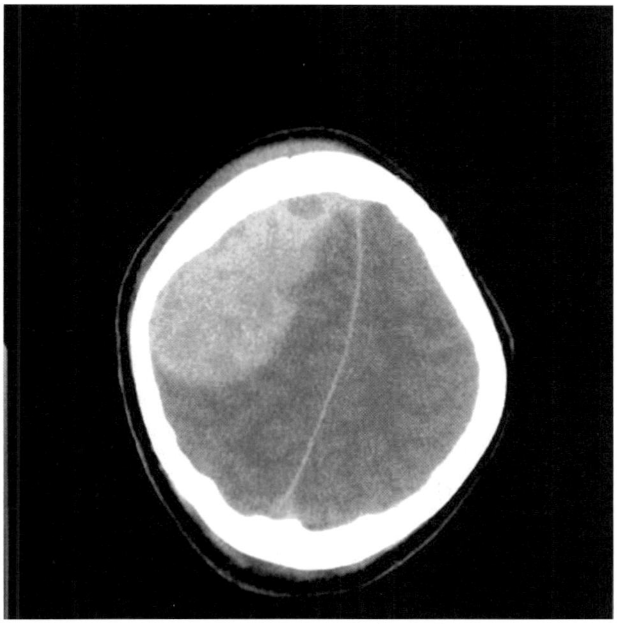

Figure 2. A CT scan demonstrating a right-sided extradural haematoma.

What is the role of the mannitol infusion?

Intravenous mannitol is used to decrease the blood volume in the brain and to decrease the brain volume due to oedema. Mannitol should not be used unless the patient is adequately resuscitated. In a haemodynamically unstable patient, mannitol may aggravate hypovolaemia and, therefore, secondary brain injury.

What is the rationale for short-term ventilation?

Hyperventilation causes cerebral vasoconstriction, thereby reducing the volume of blood in the cranial cavity and allowing room for the intracranial mass lesion. However, prolonged hyperventilation can cause cerebral ischaemia due to cerebral vasoconstriction.

Progress of the patient

- The postoperative period is uneventful. Clips were removed on the tenth postoperative day and he is discharged on day 14 postoperatively.
- Ibuprofen is prescribed for headache and phenytoin sodium as anticonvulsant treatment.
- He is advised to:
  - avoid activities such as driving, gardening, mowing, vacuuming, ironing, and loading/unloading the dishwasher, washer, or dryer till the first clinic visit;
  - refrain from alcoholic beverages;
  - return to normal activities slowly as fatigue is common;
  - follow an exercise program to gently stretch the neck and back;
  - to start with short walks and gradually increase the distance;
  - contact the primary care physician if he feels drowsy, or has balance problems, a decreased alertness, weakness of the arms or legs, increased headaches, vomiting, or severe neck pain.

What are the specific complications related to a craniotomy?

Specific complications include:

- Stroke.
- Seizures.
- Cerebral oedema.
- CSF leak, which may require repair.
- Loss of mental functions.
- Permanent brain damage with associated disabilities.

Suggested reading

1. National Institute for Health and Clinical Excellence. Head injury: triage, assessment, investigation and early management of head injury in infants, children and adults. NICE, 2007: 56.
2. Scottish Intercollegiate Guidelines Network. Early management of patients with a head injury. SIGN, 2000: 46.
3. Lane PL, Skoretz TG, Doig G, Girotti MJ. Intracranial pressure monitoring and outcomes after traumatic brain injury. *Can J Surg* 2000; 43(6): 406.

Self-assessment

Q1
EMQ

a. 4.
b. 6.
c. 10.
d. 7.
e. 11.
f. 13.

Select the Glasgow Coma Score for the case scenarios described below.

1. A young man is admitted following an assault. He screams, appears confused when spoken to, does not follow commands, moves all 4 limbs, localises to pain and opens his eyes spontaneously.
2. A 45-year-old farmer is admitted following a fall from a tree. He is haemodynamically stable and does not make any noise. Eye opening is not observed to painful stimuli but he withdraws his arm when pinched.

3. Two hours following a road crash the following findings are observed in a 23-year-old man: he does not open his eyes, there is a flexor response to a painful squeeze and an inappropriate response to verbal commands.

Q2 EMQ

a. Ventilation.
b. CT scan of brain, neck, thorax and abdomen.
c. Head injury observation.
d. Mannitol.

Select the most appropriate next step from above for the case scenarios described below.

1. A 21-year-old male is admitted with trauma to the right side of his head. He opens his eyes only to painful stimuli and withdraws from painful stimuli. He makes incomprehensible sounds. The RR is 26/minute. The pulse oximeter reads 88%. The right pupil is dilated.
2. A 45-year-old male is admitted following a fall from a tree. He is haemodynamically normal, conscious, a little confused, opens his eyes to commands and localises pain. According to relatives, he could not be roused for 15 minutes following the fall.

Q3 SBA

A 21-year-old male is seen following an assault on the right side of his head. He is haemodynamically normal. He opens his eyes only to painful stimuli. He withdraws from painful stimuli. The only verbal responses are incomprehensible sounds.

Which of the following is he likely to have?

a. Extradural haematoma.
b. Subdural haematoma.
c. Intracerebral haematoma.
d. Subarachnoid bleed.
e. Diffuse axonal injury.
f. Any of above.

Q4 True/False

a. Changes in the GCS are an indicator of the response to therapy.
b. The side on which the dilated pupil is located indicates the side of the intracaranial mass lesion.
c. Intracranial pressure monitoring is shown to improve the outcome of patients with severe head injuries.
d. Hypotension may alter the GCS independently of the brain injury.
e. Patients with a GCS below 8 are considered for ventilation.

Answers overleaf

Self-assessment answers

Q1 1. (f), 2. (b), 3. (d).

Q2 1. (a), 2. (b).

Explanatory notes

1. The clinical picture is one of an expanding intracranial mass lesion. He has arterial hypoxaemia. Immediate ventilation before surgery will reduce the severity of secondary head injury.

2. This patient's GCS is 12. However, he lost consciousness immediately after the injury. He requires a CT scan to exclude an early intracranial mass lesion.

Q3 (f).

Explanatory notes

Physical signs or the GCS do not indicate the precise nature of the head injury.

Q4 a. (T), b. (T), c. (T), d. (T), e. (T).

Chapter 18

Major burns

Learning objectives

- To learn the initial assessment and resuscitation of patients with major burns.
- To appreciate the importance of upper airway burns.
- To be familiar with the assessment and management of burn wounds.
- To learn the systemic effects and complications of major burns.

Case scenario

A 71-year-old man is admitted to the accident and emergency department with burns. He has been rescued from a house fire. The victim was found unconscious in the upstairs bedroom of a house. His past medical history is not known.

His pulse rate is 114/minute, BP is 140/75mm Hg and RR is 30/minute. The pulse oximeter records an O_2 saturation of 88% with the face mask.

Carbon deposits are seen on his face and in other exposed parts. He has blisters on his face. His eyelids are swollen. Burns involving the entire circumference of his left upper arm, left leg, back of the chest and the abdomen are seen, involving approximately 50% of the total body surface area (TBSA).

He does not respond to verbal stimuli but responds to painful stimuli with groans.

The most likely clinical diagnosis: major burns with evidence of inhalational injury to the upper airway.

What is the next step?

- Primary and secondary surveys are carried out using the ABC approach (see Chapter 16).
- This patient has major burns, with evidence of inhalational injuries and possible carbon monoxide poisoning.
- He is immediately intubated and ventilated. Fluid resuscitation is commenced using the Parkland formula.

Circumstances of the injury (house fire), the age of the patient and the extent of burns indicate a high probability of pulmonary complications.

He has a high risk of thermal damage to his upper airway because he was found unconscious in a closed space fire.

The presence of carbon deposits and blisters on his face and the reduced arterial oxygen saturation also indicate the possibility of upper airway burns.

Carbon monoxide (CO) poisoning can cause hypoxia because CO has a 240-fold greater affinity for haemoglobin than O_2. Therefore, early ventilation is important to prevent hypoxaemic injury to the vital organs. A carboxyhaemoglobin level of greater than 30% may indicate a risk of significant central nervous system dysfunction which may be permanent. Therefore, if available, all patients injured in closed space fires should have their carboxyhaemoglobin levels measured.

What is the Parkland formula?

Total volume for 24 hours =
3-4ml x body weight in Kg x % of burn.

Half the total volume is infused in 8 hours; the remainder within the next 16 hours. In children weighing less than 10Kg the formula is:

2-3ml x body weight in Kg x % burn area
(the fluid should contain 5% dextrose).

Clinical points

- Airway compromise is an immediate life-threatening complication of burns.
- Burn patients can acquire other injuries, which must be recognised and managed concurrently; hence the reason to perform primary and secondary surveys.
- Fluid resuscitation is the most important component of resuscitation after correcting the airway because cutaneous burns cause accelerated fluid loss.
- Patients with a burn size of less than 15% can be resuscitated with oral fluids.
- A burn size of more than 20% will cause a systemic response leading to hypovolaemia and, therefore, intravenous fluid replacement is required. Colloids, e.g. gelofusine, are generally avoided during the first 24 hours because of increased capillary permeability.
- Adequacy of fluid replacement is gauged by hourly urine output or CVP measurement.
- Calculating the burn area is based on the 'rule of nine'. The palm of the patient's hand represents approximately 1% of the patient's total body surface.

What signs would suggest potential airway involvement?

- Facial and upper body burns.
- Carbonaceous sputum.
- Dry, red or blistered oropharynx.
- Circumferential neck burns.

Progress of the patient

- The depth of the burn wound is assessed, photographed and recorded in the chart.
- No joint surfaces are involved.
- No circumferential burns are present.
- The burned area is cleaned with N saline.
- Carbonaceous deposits are removed. Blisters are not disturbed.
- All burn surfaces are dressed with two layers of antibacterial impregnated vaseline gauze, generous absorptive dressings and retention dressings to protect the wounds.
- The patient is ventilated in an isolated area on the HDU.
- Ranitidine 150mg IV b.d. is administered.
- Nasogastric feeding is commenced.

The skin, being the largest organ of the body, plays an important role in maintaining fluid balance. Loss of this protective barrier results in accelerated fluid loss. The injured tissue releases mediators such as prostaglandins which cause oedema and increased capillary permeability.

Interstitial oedema can occur not only in the injured area but also in distant soft tissues resulting in significant 'third space' fluid loss due to the mediator effect. This is referred to as a systemic inflammatory response. Therefore, patients with major burns will soon develop hypoperfusion of the vital organs. This hypovolaemic injury is aggravated by mediators, which leads to multiple organ dysfunction.

Loss of the protective barrier results in exposure to microbes. As a result secondary infection of the burnt surface will soon follow.

Gastric and duodenal 'stress' ulcers may develop in burn patients. Early feeding is recommended to improve nutrition, prevent stress ulcers and minimise the development of nosocomial pneumonia by inhibiting bacterial overgrowth. H2 receptor blockers are useful in preventing the occurence of stress ulers.

How is the depth of the burn wound assessed?

Depth of the wound is difficult to assess soon after the injury. This is generally classified as partial thickness and full thickness. A comparison is shown in Table 1.

What are the principles of local treatment of burn wounds?

The main objective is to keep the wound moist, clean and protected from infection. The blisters are not disturbed unless there is evidence of infection or

Table 1. Comparison of partial and full thickness burns.

	Colour	Skin texture	Pain sensation
Partial thickness	Pink - red +/- blisters	Oedematous	Present
Full thickness	Dark red/ white, brown or black	Leathery	Absent

pain. Debridement of devitalised tissue is deferred until the tissue is dried and easily removable. This will take at least 3-5 days. Early debridement is indicated when a joint surface is involved.

In most specialised units, the initial burn cleaning is done with normal saline. A generous amount of topical antimicrobial preparations such as sliver sulphadiazine is applied. The wound is then covered with non-adherent dressings such as antibacterial-impregnated vaseline gauze and absorptive dressings. This is supported by retention dressings such as tubigrip or a crepe bandage to hold the dressing firmly in place.

Hydrocolloids, calcium alginates and synthetic skin substitutes are some of the alternative dressings used by specialised burns units depending on the need.

Generally the dressings are changed after 48 hours. In some units intravenous ketamine (1-2mg/Kg) is commonly used as an analgesic during dressings. Antibiotics are usually not indicated unless there is evidence of systemic sepsis.

Progress of the patient

- Reassessment is done on the fifth day.
- The circumferential burn area on the left upper arm is excised and a split skin graft is performed. The skin is obtained from the unburned anterior abdominal wall. The rest of the burn area shows evidence of partial thickness burns with skin islets.
- Ventilation is discontinued on the fifth day.
- Physiotherapy is commenced.
- Local wound dressings are continued under ketamine anaesthesia.

What are the complications of major burns?

Complications of burns can be classified based upon the time of onset as early, intermediate and late.

They can also be classified into systems, because of the multisystem involvement of the condition as follows:

- Pulmonary:
  - respiratory failure;
  - adult respiratory distress syndrome (ARDS);
  - pneumonia.
- Renal:
  - acute tubular necrosis due to hypovolaemia and/or myoglobinuria.
- Gastrointestinal:
  - stomach and duodenal ulcers due to decreased mucosal defences as a result of a decrease in splanchnic blood flow;
  - hypoperfusion can also result in a calculous cholecystitis, acute pancreatitis and hepatic dysfunction.
- Cardiovascular:
  - deep venous thrombosis;
  - acute bacterial endocarditis;
  - suppurative thrombophlebitis.
- Ophthalmic:
  - corneal ulcerations;
  - eyelid problems due to contracture.
- Neurological:
  - delirium;
  - altered mental status. Hypoxia, metabolic abnormalities, the psychological effects of trauma and the effects of disfigurement may be responsible for altered mental status.
- Infections:
  - local infections with hospital-acquired resistant bacteria;
  - nosocomial pneumonia;
  - catheter-related sepsis;
  - central line-related sepsis;
  - sinusitis;
  - ear infection.
- Musculoskeletal:
  - scarring;
  - contracture due to joint involvement.

Progress of the patient

- The split skin graft takes well. Facial blistering and swelling regresses after 1 week. The facial scarring is assessed by the plastic surgeons. Fortunately the facial burns are superficial and no deep burns are present across joint surfaces. He is discharged home on physiotherapy after 3 weeks.

Clinical points

- With burns, contracture usually appears when the scar line is vertical to the natural tension lines, as in scars over a joint.

Suggested reading

1. Papini R. ABC of burns: management of burn injuries of various depths. *BMJ* 2004; 329: 158-60.

Self-assessment

Q1
EMQ

a. Insertion of a CVP line.
b. Insertion of a wide-bore cannula and intravenous hydration.
c. Endotracheal intubation and ventilation.
d. Protective covering of the burn area with dressings.
e. Intravenous antibiotics.
f. Intravenous morphine.

Select the most appropriate next step in the management of the patient for the case scenarios described below.

1. A 71-year-old man has been rescued, having been found unconscious from a house fire. Carbon deposits and blisters are seen on his face. The eyelids are swollen. He responds to painful stimuli. His pulse rate is 114/minute, BP is 140/75mm Hg and RR is 30/minute. The pulse oximeter records an O_2 saturation of 90% with the face mask.
2. A 55-year-old man has been rescued from a house fire with TBSA burns of 40%. He is in severe pain. He is conscious and rational. His pulse rate is 114/minute, BP is 140/75mm Hg and RR is 24/minute.
3. A 65-year-old farmer is admitted with 45% burns. He is conscious and rational. His pulse rate is 114/minute, BP is 140/75mm Hg and RR is 24/minute.

Q2
EMQ

a. Decreased mucosal defences.
b. Third space loss.
c. Upper airway burns.
d. Closed space fire.
e. Myoglobinuria.

Select the most appropriate item from above for the clinical conditions related to burns described below.

1. Carbon deposits on the face.
2. Stress ulcers.
3. Hypotension.
4. Renal failure.
5. Carbon monoxide poisoning.

Q3
SBA

An elderly lady is rescued from a fire with facial burns. Her eyes and lips are swollen. She looks drowsy and is unable to speak. Her pulse rate is 120/minute, BP is 100/75mmHg and RR is 32/min. The pulse oximeter records an O_2 saturation of 88% with oxygen delivered via the face mask at 10L/minute.

What is the most appropriate next step in the immediate management of this patient?

a. Insertion of a central venous cannula.
b. Endotracheal intubation and ventilation.
c. Dressing of burn area with silver sulphadiazine.
d. Intravenous antibiotics.
e. Intravenous morphine.

Q4
True/False

Major burns can be complicated by:

a. Peptic ulceration.
b. Acute tubular necrosis.
c. Acute pancreatitis.
d. Acute cholecystitis.
e. Myoglobinuria.

Answers overleaf

Self-assessment answers

Q1 1. (c), 2. (f), 3. (b).

Explanatory notes

1. This patient has evidence of upper airway burns from a closed space fire. He is hypoxaemic. It is very likely that he has upper airway burns and carbon monoxide poisoning. Immediate intubation to establish and protect the airway, and ventilation to treat the hypoxaemia are the most appropriate next steps.

2. This patient has significant burns and is in severe pain. He may develop neurogenic shock. Burn pain can be very severe and the most appropriate next step is to treat him with intravenous morphine.

3. The elderly farmer with 45% burns is likely to have significant fluid loss. Intravenous fluid administration is the most appropriate next step.

Q2 1. (c), 2. (a), 3. (b), 4. (e). 5. (d).

Q3 (b).

Q4 a. (T), b. (T), c. (T), d (T), e. (T).

Chapter 19

Groin hernia

Learning objectives

- To learn the clinical presentation of inguinal and femoral herniae.
- To recollect the anatomical landmarks of the types of groin herniae.
- To understand the options for hernia repair.

Case scenario

A 40-year-old man presents with a history of pain in the left groin of 12 hours' duration. The pain developed when he was lifting a bag of fertiliser while working on the farm. He recalls having a slight swelling which used to appear on and off in the past. He has no significant past medical problems or a past history of surgery.

Examination reveals an obese, fit looking man. Cardiovascular and abdominal examinations are unremarkable. Examination of the right inguinal region is normal. On the left side, there is a 3cm x 2cm non-erythematous, tender swelling at the medial part of the left groin crease in the region of the pubic tubercle

Careful examination reveals that the neck of the lump is just above the inguinal ligament but the anatomy is difficult due to groin fat. The lump is not reducible. A gentle attempt at reduction is met with discomfort. The scrotal sac is normal and both testes feel normal.

Laboratory investigations reveal normal haematological and biochemical parameters.

An abdominal X-ray is normal.

The most likely clinical diagnosis: incarcerated left inguinal hernia.

In the groin, the inguinal ligament provides a dividing line structurally between inguinal herniae and femoral herniae.

Inguinal herniae are further divided into direct and indirect types in relation to the inferior epigastric vessels. The inferior epigastric vein and artery form the medial margin of the internal ring (Figure 1).

An indirect hernia enters the internal ring traversing the inguinal canal and appears at the external ring. It exits through the external ring and may extend into the scrotal sac. Because the inferior epigastric vessels are related to the medial border of the internal ring, the hernial sac of an indirect inguinal hernia is found lateral to the inferior epigastric vessels.

The weakest point in the inguinal region is the Hasselbach triangle. This is defined by the free edge of the conjoint tendon superomedially, inguinal ligament inferiorly and inferior epigastric vessels laterally. In this triangle, the peritoneum and transversalis fascia are the only supportive coverings on the posterior aspect of the inguinal canal. As shown in Figure 1, direct inguinal herniae protrude through this area of potential weakness. This potential weakness is present in every human from birth.

A second site of weakness is the stretched and weakened internal inguinal ring which occurs when intra-abdominal pressure pushes the contents through the internal ring. The site of the internal ring again is a potential weak point. During embryological development this was the passage where the testis descended down to the scrotal sac dragging its blood supply all the way from the abdominal cavity.

These two sites should be reinforced when repair is carried out for a inguinal hernia.

Femoral herniae appear via the femoral canal which is the medial compartment of the femoral sheath and appears out of the femoral ring (Figure 2).

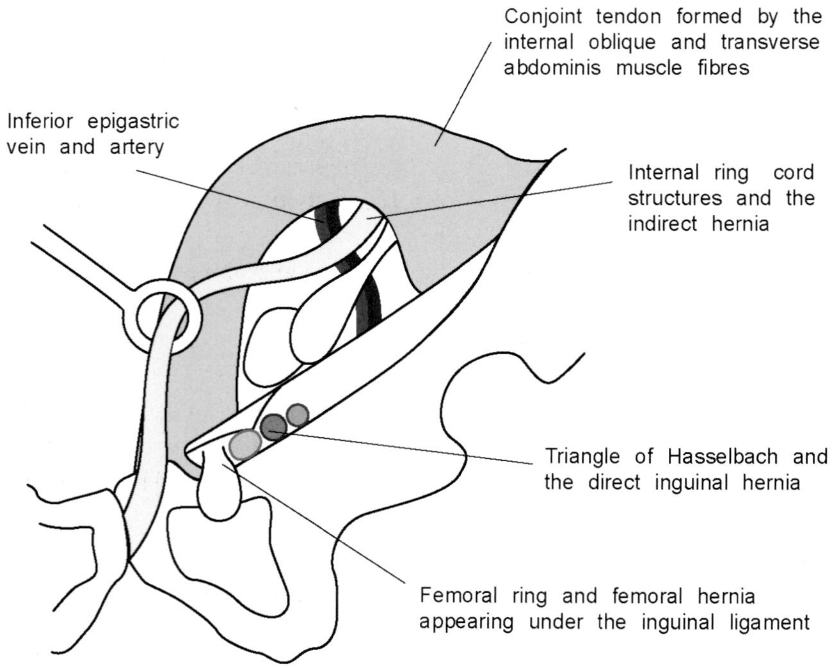

Figure 1. The surgical anatomy of the inguinal region.

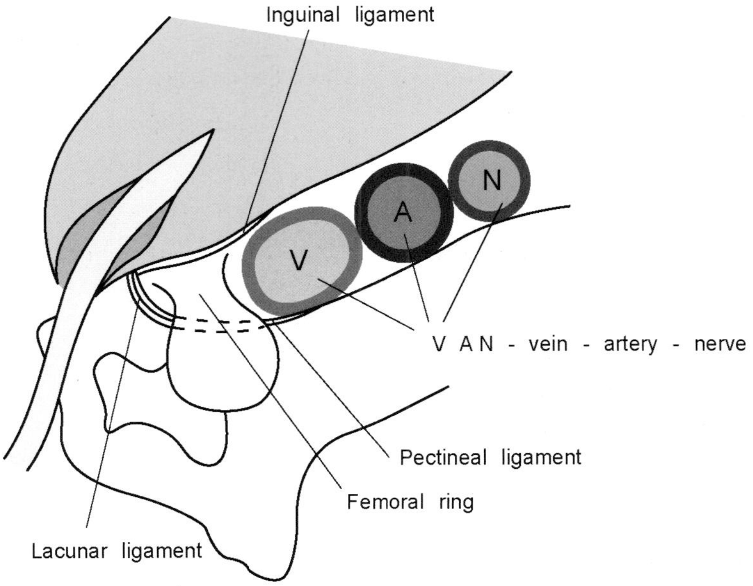

Figure 2. The surgical anatomy of the femoral region.

The femoral ring is defined medially by the lacunar ligament, anteriorly by the inguinal ligament, posteriorly by the pectineal ligament and laterally by the femoral vein. At surgery the lateral margin of the neck of a femoral hernia is exposed with care to prevent accidental injury to the femoral vein. Because the inguinal ligament is attached to the pubic tubercle, the femoral hernia is always below the inguinal ligament, and below and lateral to the pubic tubercle. An indirect inguinal hernia appears out through the external ring and therefore the point of appearance is above and medial to the pubic tubercle and above the inguinal ligament.

A sizable direct inguinal hernia may confuse a student because it may overlap this region.

Most patients with inguinal herniae are aware of a swelling in the region. The swelling is more prominent on standing or during physical activity and is usually reducible on lying down. It may cause intermittent groin pain or a feeling of heaviness.

In contrast, a femoral hernia may not be noticed by the patient because of their relatively small size. This is especially so in obese patients when the swelling may be hidden in the groin fat.

The sudden onset of a painful groin mass as is in this patient suggests incarceration of a hernia. A muscle injury or a muscle haematoma should be considered in the differential diagnosis. Patients who are on anticoagulants are more likely to develop such haematomas.

An enlarged lymph node in the groin may be confused with an irreducible femoral hernia. It is therefore always important to check the genitalia and the anal region when considering a diagnosis of a femoral hernia.

Clinical points

- Femoral herniae appear below the inguinal ligament and below and lateral to the pubic tubercle.
- The neck of an indirect inguinal hernia appears above the inguinal ligament, and above and medial to the pubic tubercle.
- Indirect inguinal herniae traverse through the inguinal canal and may extend to the scrotum.
- A direct hernia appears through the Hasselbach triangle, medial to the internal ring.
- Because femoral herniae are usually small there may be minimal or no symptoms and acute incarceration may be the initial presentation.

What is meant by incarceration?

In all abdominal wall herniae the abdominal contents protrude through a defect in the abdominal wall. The contents may be omentum, small bowel, colon, bladder or any other organ such as the ovary or appendix. Small bowel and omentum are commonly found in the hernial sac. When the contents are reducible the hernia is referred to as a reducible hernia.

Sometimes the contents can become adherent in the sac. This is called incarceration. When this happens suddenly the sac can become tender. Strangulation occurs when the blood supply to the trapped contents becomes compromised, which leads to ischaemia and necrosis. Ischaemic omentum may become gangrenous and form an abscess.

Intestinal obstruction can occur in an incarcerated or strangulated hernia. However, a part of the bowel wall can occasionally become trapped at the neck of a hernia without causing obstruction to the lumen. This is called Richter's hernia.

What is the next step?

- The patient is taken to the operating theatre as an emergency.
- A broad-spectrum antibiotic (e.g. cefuroxime) is given at induction and also a dose of low-molecular-weight heparin because this patient is obese.
- Under general anaesthesia, a transverse incision is made over the swelling. An indirect inguinal hernia with a tight neck is identified. The cord structures look oedematous. The sac is dissected out and opened. The oedematous omentum and congested small bowel are released from the attachments and reduced to the abdomen. The bowel appears viable. The sac is excised and the defect is closed by inserting a mesh (Lichtenstein operation).
- The patient returns home after 48 hours.

What is the rationale for using a mesh in the repair of an inguinal hernia?

Historically the most popular technique for the repair of an inguinal hernia was the Bassini repair where the conjoint tendon is approximated to the inguinal ligament by non-absorbable sutures. Approximation of tissue leads to tension which is thought to be the main reason for recurrence following surgery. Placement of non-absorbable mesh to cover the defect instead of approximating tissue avoids the problem of tension. Many studies have consistently shown lower recurrence rates with mesh placement. The placement of mesh has become the treatment of choice for the repair of inguinal herniae.

Mesh may be placed by an open technique under local (often with the addition of sedation) or general anaesthesia (GA). It can also be placed laparoscopically using a preperitoneal or intraperitoneal approach under GA. The majority of hernia repairs are suitable for repair as day cases.

In the open technique the mesh is placed on the posterior wall of the inguinal canal, the internal ring is reconstructed and the mesh is tagged by interrupted sutures.

In the laparoscopic technique the hernia is reduced and the mesh is placed to cover the defect. Connective tissue grows into the mesh and the mesh becomes incorporated into the tissue.

Complications of mesh placement include seroma formation, infection and displacement. Chronic groin pain is reported in a significant number of patients but is rarely an important problem. Whilst gaining informed consent these issues must be discussed.

Progress of the patient

- The patient is discharged on the first postoperative day with follow-up arrangements.
- Diclofenac and paracetamol are prescribed for pain.
- The basic principle is that he can resume what he is comfortable doing in his own time. As a guide he is advised:
  - to rest for 24 hours;
  - to refrain from strenuous activity for 2 weeks;
  - that he may climb stairs;
  - that he may assume sexual activity when he can tolerate this without significant discomfort;
  - to return to work in 1-2 weeks (clerical work) and 4 weeks (manual labour);
  - that he can drive when it feels comfortable;
  - that he should not drive while on narcotic analgesics if found to be necessary;
  - not to consume alcohol when he is on medication.

Suggested reading

1. Bisgaard T, Bay-Nielsen M, Kehlet H. Re-recurrence after operation for recurrent inguinal hernia. A nationwide 8-year follow-up study on the role of type of repair. *Ann Surg* 2008; 247(4): 707-11
2. Zollinger R, Jr. Classification systems for groin hernias. *Surgical Clinics of North America* 2003; 83: 1053-63.

Self-assessment

Q1
EMQ

a. Indirect inguinal hernia.
b. Strangulated inguinal hernia.
c. Obstructed hernia.
d. Incarcerated femoral hernia.

Select the most likely clinical diagnosis from the conditions mentioned above for the case scenarios described below.

1. An elderly female presents with a tender, irreducible swelling below the inguinal ligament and lateral to the pubic tubercle.
2. A 65-year-old morbidly obese female presents with acute small bowel obstruction. She has had abdominal pain and vomiting for 4 days and had been treated for gastroenteritis by the primary care physician before the groin swelling was noticed. She has no past history of abdominal surgery. She has a tense, tender, irreducible swelling in the groin with no skin erythema over it.
3. An 80-year-old male who lives alone is brought in with a large, tender, irreducible swelling in the right groin. He complains of nausea and vomiting. He looks unwell. The skin over the lump is shiny and erythematous with surrounding cellulitis. He has not passed faeces or flatus for 3 days and his abdomen is distended.

Q2
SBA

A surgical registrar has explored the groin of an obese male who presented with an irreducible, painful tender swelling in the right groin. A black loop of small bowel is found densely adherent to the neck of a femoral hernia and while trying to release it a perforation of the gangrenous bowel occurred because of limited space.

What is the most appropriate next step?

a. Resect the gangrenous bowel, anastomose the ends of the normal bowel and repair the hernia with a polypropylene mesh.
b. Resect the gangrenous bowel, anastomose the ends of the normal bowel and repair the hernia with non-absorbable sutures.
c. Resect the gangrenous bowel, anastomose the ends of the normal bowel, close the hernial sac without performing a repair and plan for a laparoscopic repair at a future date.
d. Perform a mini-laparotomy, resect the small bowel, anastomose the two ends of normal bowel and repair the femoral hernia with non-absorbable sutures.
e. Perform a mini-laparotomy, resect the small bowel, exteriorize the two ends of the bowel as end ileostomies and repair the femoral hernia with non-absorbable sutures.

Q3
True/False

a. Femoral hernia is the most common type of groin hernia encountered in females.
b. Femoral hernia is more common in females than males.
c. Recurrences after primary repair of inguinal hernia is less with mesh placement as compared with non-mesh techniques.
d. When a recurrence occurs following primary repair of an inguinal hernia the common site for the recurrence is the medial end of the defect.
e. The risk of re-recurrence is higher compared with the risk of recurrence after primary inguinal hernia repair.

Answers overleaf

Self-assessment answers

Q1 1. (d), 2. (c), 3. (b).

Explanatory notes

2. In morbidly obese patients it may be difficult to distinguish inguinal from femoral herniae. This will not affect the clinical decision making in this patient because she has features of small bowel obstruction and therefore she needs a laparotomy and not groin exploration. The justification for this decision is that she is likely to have bowel ischaemia because of the duration of symptoms. It is not a safe practice to attempt bowel resection and anastomosis through a small groin incision in a morbidly obese patient.

3. A tense, tender irreducible groin swelling with erythema of the skin and surrounding cellulitis is suggestive of a strangulated hernia. It is unlikely to be a groin abscess because he has features of acute intestinal obstruction.

Q2 (d).

Explanatory notes

Performing a small bowel anastomosis under tension through limited access is likely to fail. The safest option is to explore through a lower midline incision, mobilise the loop gently into the peritoneal cavity and perform resection and a tensionless anastomosis. Because the bowel perforation has occurred in the groin wound it is best to avoid a mesh repair.

Q3 a. (F), b. (T), c. (T), d. (T) e. (T).

Chapter 20

Scrotal swelling

Learning objectives

- To learn to arrive at a clinical diagnosis of a patient presenting with a scrotal swelling.

Case scenario

A 72-year-old retired farmer decides to seek advice from his primary care physician for a longstanding scrotal swelling because of increasing discomfort. The primary care physician refers him to the surgical clinic.

The patient has noticed that the right side of his scrotum has been larger than the left for 2 years. This has slowly grown in size to the extent that he is feeling heaviness in the swelling and is finding it difficult to wear his underpants.

His past medical history is significant for hypertension for which he is on medication. He is also on aspirin.

Examination reveals a 10cm x12cm, non-tender cystic swelling involving the right side of the scrotum.

In the standing position, the swelling appears to be confined to the scrotum. The right testis is not palpable. His left scrotal sac and testis are normal.

The swelling is not transilluminable.

An abdominal examination is unremarkable.

The most likely clinical diagnosis: a right-sided vaginal hydrocele.

Other conditions to be considered in the differential diagnosis of a scrotal lump include an inguinoscrotal hernia, an epididymal cyst, a spermatocele and cancer of the testis.

The answers to the following questions will differentiate the conditions mentioned above.

Can I get above the lump?

If the answer is yes, this excludes an inguinoscrotal hernia from the differential diagnosis because the hernia descends down from the external ring and therefore on examination, one cannot get above the swelling.

Can I feel the testis?

If the answer is yes, this excludes a vaginal hydrocele. A hydrocele is a collection of fluid around the testis and therefore the testis should not be palpable. The exception is a small hydrocele where it may be still possible to palpate the testis.

If the testis can be felt, does it feel like a normal testis or an abnormal testis?

If it feels like a normal testis then the swelling could be an epididymal cyst or a spermatocele.

If the testis is normal, is the swelling transilluminable?

If yes, then this is an epididymal cyst; if no, then this is a spermatocele.

If the testis feels abnormal (hard, craggy), testicular cancer needs to be excluded.

An epididymal cyst contains clear fluid. At surgery it is not uncommon to see that a clinically palpable swelling contains cysts of different sizes. The clear fluid-filled cysts of different sizes make the swelling brilliantly transilluminable. The appearance is described as a 'Chinese lantern'.

A spermatocele contains sperm and therefore is not transilluminable.

This patient has a cystic scrotal lump confined to the right scrotal sac which indicates that he has fluid around the testis. This is why his testis is not palpable. However, it is expected that the light will shine through the fluid, to produce the physical sign, transillumination, which is not elicited in this patient. This may be because the fluid might be turbid or the wall of the hydrocele sac may be too thick to transmit light. This is sometimes seen with longstanding hydroceles. Like this farmer it is not uncommon to see elderly patients who do not seek treatment for a considerable length of time because of the absence of any significant symptoms related to the scrotal swelling.

What is the next step?

- An ultrasound scan of the scrotum is obtained. This confirms a thick-walled hydrocele. The testis is normal.

Progress of the patient

- The patient undergoes a hydrocelectomy.
- Under general anaesthesia the sac is opened through a transverse incision, fluid is drained out and the excess sac is excised. Careful haemostasis is obtained, especially as the patient is on aspirin.

Some surgeons would discontinue aspirin about a week prior to the procedure as it increases the risk of postoperative haematoma formation. The procedure can be performed under general, local or spinal anaesthesia.

Clinical points

- Haematoma formation and infection are two recognised complications associated with a hydrocelectomy.

Progress of the patient

- The immediate postoperative period is uneventful.
- Some residual swelling in the scrotum with skin discolouration is noted and the patient accepts the explanation that this is not an unusual finding following surgery for hydroceles. He is reassured that this will regress with time.

Suggested reading

1. Haynes J. Inguinal and scrotal disorders. *Surgical Clinics of North America* 2006; 86(2): 371-81.

Self-assessment

Q1
EMQ

a. Cancer of the testis.
b. Haematocele.
c. Thick-walled hydrocele.
d. Spermatocele.
e. Scrotal hernia.
f. Epididymal cyst.

Select the most likely clinical diagnosis from the conditions mentioned above for the case scenarios described below.

1. Cystic scrotal lump, cannot get above the swelling, non-transilluminable.
2. Cystic scrotal lump, can get above the swelling, testis can be felt, markedly transilluminable.
3. Firm tender lump, testis cannot be felt, non-transilluminable.
4. Hard non-tender irregular lump in the scrotal sac with thickening of the cord.
5. Cystic scrotal lump, can get above the swelling, testis cannot be felt, non-transilluminable.
6. Cystic scrotal lump, can get above the swelling, testis can be felt, non-transilluminable.

Q2
SBA

A surgical registrar is requested to perform a hydrocelectomy. At surgery under general anaesthesia he finds that the patient has a thick-walled hydrocele sac, some fluid in the sac and a vascular testicular mass which has not been detected pre-operatively. The mass appears suspicious of a cancer.

What is the most appropriate next step?

a. Biopsy the lump and close the skin.
b. Perform an orchidectomy.
c. Remove the fluid and do a hydrocelectomy.
d. Call the surgeon to theatre for clinical judgement.
e. Do not proceed and close the skin only.

Q3
True/False

Causative factors of a hydrocele include:

a. Testicular cancer.
b. Filarial infection.
c. Trauma.
d. Tuberculous infection in the testis.
e. Prostate cancer.

Answers overleaf

Self-assessment answers

Q1 1. (e), 2. (f), 3. (b), 4. (a), 5. (c), 6. (d).

Q2 (d).

Explanatory notes

The next step in this rare clinical scenario has considerable clinical and medico-legal implications. Experience and expertise are required to handle this situation with regard to further treatment and for communication with the patient and relatives. It is important for the trainee to appreciate the need for the surgeon in charge of the patient or at least another senior experienced surgeon to become involved at this stage and to adhere to best practice principles. It is also important to accurately document the details of the findings and the sequence of events carried out.

Q3 a. (T), b. (T), c. (T), d. (T), e. (F).

Chapter 21

Ureteric colic

Learning objectives

- To learn the initial assessment of a patient presenting with ureteric colic.
- To learn the diagnostic and management options of patients with suspected upper urinary tract obstruction with infection.

Case scenario

A 45-year-old man is admitted to the emergency room with severe abdominal pain of 3 hours' duration. Pain commenced as an ache in the left upper abdomen and left loin area but soon increased to an excruciating pain radiating to the lower abdomen and scrotum. He has an urge to urinate but can only void a small quantity of red-coloured urine. About a month ago he had a mild but similar episode that responded to paracetamol.

He denies any past history of urinary problems.

He has no other medical problems. He drinks socially during weekends and smokes about 10 cigarettes a day for the last 10 years.

On examination he is in severe pain, his temperature is 38.5°C, pulse rate is 86/minute and RR is 20/minute. He is pleading for pain relief.

Examination reveals some tenderness in the left hypochondrium and in the left renal angle but the interpretation is difficult because he is in severe pain.

The most likely clinical diagnosis: left-sided ureteric colic with possible sepsis.

The severity, location and radiation of pain is characteristic of ureteric colic. The most likely clinical diagnosis, therefore, is a left ureteric stone. Severe pain is due to ureteric peristalsis acting against the obstruction and also due to distension of the upper urinary tract. The macroscopic haematuria is indicative of an erosive lesion of the ureteric mucosa due to the passage of a stone.

Acute pancreatitis, acute diverticulitis and a leaking abdominal aortic aneurysm require consideration in the differential diagnosis.

What is the next step?

- The patient is given 10mg of morphine intravenously.
- Urine full report - proteins +, red cells field full.
- A urine sample is sent for culture.
- Blood culture - sent.
- WCC 18,000/mm^3.
- Blood urea - normal.
- S amylase - normal.
- S creatinine - normal.
- S calcium and uric acid - normal.
- X-ray KUB - there is a shadow in line with the left ureter at the level of the 3rd lumbar vertebra.
- A broad-spectrum antibiotic (e.g. ciprofloxacin 500mg IV) is administered.
- An intravenous infusion is started with N saline 8-hourly and urine output is closely monitored.

Pyrexia, renal angle tenderness and the high white cell count indicate the onset of upper urinary tract infection. It is possible that he has an obstructive lesion in the upper urinary system. He may need urgent decompression. Missed upper urinary tract obstruction is associated with a significant assault on renal function.

Progress of the patient

- An urgent ultrasound scan is arranged.
- The pain responds to IV morphine.
- His temperature comes down to baseline but after 4 hours he develops another spike of 39.5°C with a chill.
- The ultrasound scan shows obstructive gross hydronephrosis and a distended upper ureter on the left side. The right kidney is normal.

Clinical points

- Ultrasound is the imaging of choice to determine the presence of hydronephrosis in many centres.

Why is an urgent intravenous urogram (IVU) or contrast CT urogram not performed?

This patient has clinical and ultrasound evidence of significant upper tract obstruction. Renal dysfunction may result in non-excretion of the contrast; hence a nephrogram may not show up anything.

There is a risk of contrast nephropathy in the presence of obstruction. Alternatively, a non-contrast CT urogram (stone protocol) may be used. A helical CT scan without contrast is replacing X-ray of the kidney, ureter and bladder (KUB) as the first step in radiological evaluation of the urinary system in some centres.

Magnetic resonance imaging (MRI) is highly sensitive for urinary tract obstruction, but it cannot differentiate functional dilatation from anatomical obstruction.

This patient requires urgent decompression of the obstructed left kidney. The overall clinical picture and results of investigations indicate a significant upper urinary tract obstruction with sepsis.

What is the next step?

- International normalised ratio (INR) 1.3.
- A percutaneous nephrostomy is performed under ultrasound guidance. 100ml of turbid fluid is drained. Urinary drainage is established. A specimen is sent for culture. The broad-spectrum antibiotic (e.g. ciprofloxacin 500mg IV b.d.) is continued.
- Blood culture grows *Escherichia coli* which is sensitive to ciprofloxacin.
- The temperature subsides with percutaneous drainage.

What is a percutaneous nephrostomy?

Percutaneous nephrostomy is a procedure which is used to decompress an obstructed renal collecting system. The commonest indication is to relieve urinary obstruction secondary to calculi. Frequently, the obstructed system becomes infected, and antibiotics are unable to penetrate the kidney when the purulent material is not drained.

The procedure involves the placement of a tube into the renal collecting system under ultrasound or X-ray guidance to drain the infected urine. A sample is collected for culture. Dye is injected and the images often demonstrate the level and cause of obstruction.

A percutaneous nephrostomy may be a life-saving procedure for patients who have septicaemia due to pyonephrosis.

Complications associated with percutaneous nephrostomy include bleeding, septicaemia, and injury to the kidney or adjacent vessels and organs.

An alternative treatment is cystoscopy and insertion of a JJ stent under general anaesthesia. Under fluoroscopic guidance, a silicone tube is positioned past the stone to be curled up in the kidney and the lower end remains in the bladder. The patient can undergo further treatment such as extracorporeal shock wave lithotripsy (ESWL) at a later stage.

This may avoid surgery because the obstructing calculus may spontaneously pass when the oedema within the ureter subsides.

Progress of the patient

- One week after the temperature subsides, a nephrostogram is performed through the nephrostomy tube (Figure 1).
- This shows an obstructing ureteric stone in the upper one third of the left ureter with distension of the renal collecting system.
- A JJ stent is inserted and the patient undergoes extracorporeal shock wave lithotripsy (ESWL) for stone fragmentation.

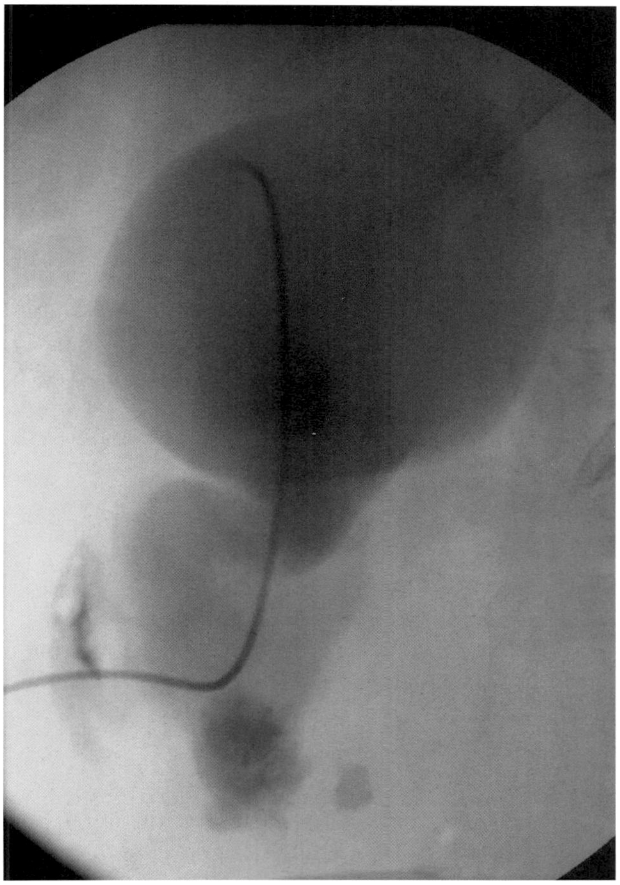

Figure 1. Nephrostogram showing a complete calculous obstruction of the left ureter. ***Reproduced with permission from Dr John Scally, Consultant Radiologist, Leighton Hospital, Crewe, UK.***

Would the position of the stone have an influence on treatment strategy?

Yes. An obstructed renal collecting system is best dealt with by percutaneous nephrostomy to drain the infected urine. Once the emergency subsides, the next step is definitive treatment of the stone disease. The best approach is the non-invasive method of ESWL. Once the stone is fragmented, small fragments can become lodged in the ureter and may cause colic or even obstruction. This is called Stein strasse. To prevent this, a JJ stent is inserted as a prophylactic measure after cystoscopy. The stent is extracted a few weeks after stone clearance.

An alternative treatment for a stone in the collecting system is percutaneous nephrolithotomy (PCNL). This technique is suitable for larger (>1.5-2cm) stones in the collecting system. Under radiological guidance, a tract to the obstructed collecting system is created. The tract is dilated to a size in order to accept a nephroscope. The stones are then fragmented and completely cleared.

Ureteric stones lodged in the ureter may also be approached via a ureteroscope. The stone is fragmented with laser or an electrohydraulic method and the small fragments are extracted with a Dormia basket which is passed from the bladder via a cystoscope. Caution is required when dealing with high ureteric stones.

More than 90% of ureteric calculi less than 0.5-0.7cm in size will pass spontaneously.

Surgical drainage of ureteric calculi is indicated in:

- Patients with unrelenting pain.
- Patients with an obstructed and infected system.
- Persistent obstruction.

Bilateral obstruction of the ureters is uncommon. When it occurs it is almost always an asymmetrical process. Irrespective of the cause of the ureteric obstruction, one ureter obstructs slowly and asymptomatically over a period of time. It is only when the second ureter is obstructed that the patient presents with renal failure, hyperkalaemia and/or acidosis. An isotope scan is very useful to identify the most viable kidney for drainage.

Clinical points

- Bilateral ureteric obstruction is almost always an asymmetrical process.
- An isotope scan is valuable to identify the most viable kidney.
- The most viable kidney is drained first.

Progress of the patient

- A repeat ultrasound and plain X-ray confirm complete disintegration and disappearance of stone fragments. The JJ stent is extracted with the cystoscope under local anaesthesia.
- Under follow-up the patient's renal function is satisfactory.
- He is strongly advised to increase his fluid intake.

Suggested reading

1. Miller NL, Lingeman JE. Management of kidney stones. *BMJ* 2007; 334: 468-72.
2. Wu H, Docimo S. Surgical management of children with urolithiasis. *Urologic Clinics of North America* 2004; 31(3): 589-94.
3. Haleblian G, Kijvikai K, de la Rosette J, Preminger G. Ureteral stenting and urinary stone management: a systematic review. *J Urol* 2008; 179(2): 424-30.

Self-assessment

Q1
EMQ

a. Percutaneous nephrostomy.
b. ESWL.
c. Ureteric stent and ESWL.
d. PCNL.
e. Expectant treatment.
f. Ureteroscopy and stone extraction.

Select the best treatment option from above for the case scenarios described below.

1. A 45-year-old male presents with right renal colic which settles the next day. He has had a similar episode 2 months ago. He is apyrexial, has normal renal function and the urine report shows no evidence of infection. His WCC is normal. An IVU shows a non-obstructing 0.5cm stone in the left lower ureter.
2. A 64-year-old man presents with a 1.5cm stone in the right renal pelvis. He is apyrexial and has a normal WCC.
3. A 45-year-old man presents with a clinical picture suggestive of a left-sided ureteric colic. His temperature is 38.5°C, pulse rate is 86/minute and RR is 20/minute. He is tender in the left renal angle. An ultrasound scan shows gross hydronephrosis of the left collecting system.
4. A 64-year-old man presents with a 3.5cm stone in the lower collecting system in the right kidney. He is apyrexial and has a normal WCC.

Q2
EMQ

a. Ureteric colic.
b. Leaking abdominal aortic aneurysm.
c. Bladder neck stone.
d. Atrophic urethritis.
e. Lower urinary tract infection.
f. Bladder tumour.
g. Pyelonephritis.

Select the most likely clinical diagnosis from the conditions mentioned above for the case scenarios described below.

1. Painless frank haematuria.
2. Painful haematuria.
3. Acute retention in a 24-year-o d man.
4. Acute retention in an 80-year-ɔld female.
5. Loin pain and fever with chi ls in a 55-year-old female.
6. Severe abdominal pain and back pain of sudden onset in an elderly patient with a tender abdomen.

Q3
SBA

A 29-year-old man is admitted with severe abdominal pain and an inability to pass urine of 12 hours' duration after a night out. He has no past history of similer episodes. He has a severe urge to urinate but can only void a few drops of red-coloured urine.

What is the most likely clinical diagnosis?

a. Bladder tumour.
b. Bladder neck stone.
c. Marion's disease (congenital bladder neck hypertrophy).
d. Prostatic cancer.
e. Urethral stricture.

Q4
True/False

The options available to drain obstructed hydronephrosis due to stone disease include:

a. Percutaneous nephrostomy.
b. Double J stenting via a cystoscope.
c. Percutaneous nephrolithotomy (PCNL).
d. Open nephrostomy.
e. Ureteroscopic electrohydraulic lithotripsy.

Answers overleaf

Self-assessment answers

Q1 1. (e), 2. (c), 3. (a), 4. (d).

Explanatory notes

4. Due to its dependent position, stones in the lower collecting system may not be effectively cleared after fragmenting with ESWL. Therefore, stones located at this site are best dealt with by PCNL.

Q2 1. (f), 2. (a), 3. (c), 4. (d), 5. (g), 6. (b).

Q3 (b).

Explanatory notes

A common cause of acute retention of urine in a young man with no history of previous episodes is a bladder stone obstructing the outflow. A severe UTI is the other common cause to consider at this age but this alternative is not given in the question.

Q4 a. (T), b. (T), c. (T), d. (T), e. (T).

Chapter 22

Bladder outflow obstruction

Learning objectives

- To learn the clinical presentation of bladder outflow obstruction.
- To learn the differential diagnosis and management of a patient with a suspected bladder outflow obstruction.

Case scenario

A 70-year-old male presents with a 6-month history of difficulty in passing urine. He complains that at the end of passing urine he feels as if he has not emptied his bladder. This has resulted in increased frequency and he wakes up about twice during the night to void. He finds it difficult to initiate the act and the stream is slow. He dribbles at the end. When he feels the urge to urinate he cannot hold for long and this has caused wetting of his underpants, especially in cold weather.

About 4 months ago he received treatment from his primary care physician for a urinary tract infection (UTI).

He denies haematuria or a history of urethral discharge.

On examination, he looks well. His vital signs and system examination are unremarkable. An abdominal examination reveals no masses. No lower limb oedema is noted.

The digital rectal examination reveals a moderately enlarged prostate gland. The surface is smooth and the consistency is soft. No nodules are felt.

The most likely clinical diagnosis: bladder outflow obstruction most likely due to benign prostatic enlargement.

This patient presents with a combination of obstructive and irritative bladder symptoms.

Obstructive symptoms are:

- Hesitancy - having to wait for the urine to start flowing.
- Poor stream.
- Double voiding (straining to urinate).
- Post-void dribbling or terminal dribbling.
- Retention of urine.

The obstructive symptoms are caused by mechanical obstruction to urine flow. The commonest cause is benign prostatic hyperplasia (BPH). The obstructive symptoms are also referred to as voiding symptoms.

This patient also has irritative symptoms. The irritative symptoms are referred to as 'storage symptoms'. These are:

- Increased frequency.
- Nocturia.
- Urgency - unable to hold after feeling the need to pass urine.
- Incontinence.
- Dysuria.
- Sense of incomplete emptying of the bladder.

The irritative symptoms are due to a combination of mechanical obstruction and the effects of obstruction. The bladder wall contracts against the longstanding obstruction which results in hypertrophy of the bladder musculature. The stagnation of urine in the bladder may lead to recurrent cystitis. These two effects are thought to be responsible for storage symptoms.

The prostate gland is an organ which is situated at the base of the bladder. The gland is considered as a reproductive organ in the male because its function is to produce ejacuate which serves as the vehicle for spermatozoa. The gland is covered with a capsule. When the male ages, the gland increases in size but the capsule restricts the outward expansion of the gland. Therefore, it enlarges inwards and upwards. The inward enlargement causes compression of the prostatic urethra as the prostatic urethra is encircled by the prostate. It also enlarges in a cephalic direction into the bladder which eventually creates a space called a post-prostatic pouch in the bladder which can accommodate a significant quantity of residual urine. This causes stagnation of urine. Pathologically the enlargement is due to epithelial and stromal hyperplasia leading to nodule formation.

What is the accepted method for assessing the severity of prostatic symptoms?

The International Prostate Symptom Score (I-PSS) is an internationally accepted score to assess the severity of prostatic symptoms. This was originally designed by the American Urological Association.

The score is based on the answers to seven questions on urinary symptoms and one question on quality of life. Patients are allowed to choose from 1 to 5 to indicate the severity of each symptom. Each answer is assigned points from 0-5. The total score ranges from 0-35 (no symptoms to severe symptoms).

The seven symptoms are:

- Incomplete emptying.
- Frequency.
- Intermittency.
- Urgency.
- Weak stream.
- Straining.
- Nocturia.

Question 8 refers to quality of life: if you were to spend the rest of your life with your symptoms as they are now, how would you feel? (0 - delighted, 6 - terrible).

A total score of 0-7 is considered as mild, 8-19 as moderate and 20-35 as severe symptoms.

Progress of the patient

- Urine is collected for a full report and culture.
- Blood urea - normal.
- S creatinine - normal.
- Prostate specific antigen (PSA) - normal.
- An abdominal ultrasound scan is performed which identifies the presence of 200ml residual urine and moderate enlargement of the prostate.

The main purpose of the initial assessment is:

- To exclude other aetiologies such as prostate cancer, bladder cancer, a benign urethral stricture and neurological diseases, e.g. Parkinson's disease.
- To identify the presence or absence of urinary tract obstruction.
- To identify any evidence of renal compromise due to obstruction.

What is prostate specific antigen (PSA)?

Prostate specific antigen is a glycoprotein produced by the prostatic cells. High levels are associated with prostate cancer. However, the PSA level can be elevated in many benign disorders such as BPH, prostatitis, UTI, after digital rectal examination, ejaculation or even after cycle riding.

If there is nodularity or changes in the consistency of the prostate on clinical examination, the measurement of PSA and a transrectal prostatic biopsy are mandatory to exclude cancer.

Many urological surgeons routinely perform PSA testing during the work-up of a patient with symptoms of bladder outflow obstruction.

What is the next step?

- He is commenced on an alpha-adrenergic receptor blocker.

Progress of the patient

- The patient responds to medical treatment.
- One year after the treatment he is referred by his primary care physician with troublesome nocturia.
- The primary care physician has performed a PSA test which is normal.
- The primary care physician has started him on a 5-alpha-reductase inhibitor. He has a good response initially but lately the symptoms have become progressive.
- He would like to know what are the other options.

The contractions of the smooth muscles in the bladder neck and prostate are mediated by alpha-adrenergic receptors. Alpha-adrenergic receptor antagonists (e.g. tamsulosin or alfuzosin) act by blocking contractions of the smooth muscle of the prostate and bladder neck. These drugs are effective within a few days and are generally well tolerated. Occasionally, they can cause hypotension, dizziness, headache, decreased erections and retrograde ejaculation (dry orgasm).

What are the other drugs used in the medical management of prostatic hyperplasia?

The other drug is an alpha-reductase inhibitor (e.g. finasteride). It acts by competitively inhibiting alpha-reductase, an enzyme that converts testosterone to dihydrotestosterone (DHT). DHT is the androgen that stimulates the development of prostate tissue. The enzyme, alpha-reductase, is found in the prostate. Therefore, the drug reduces the size of the prostate, which improves urine flow. The alpha-reductases take about 3-6 weeks to have an effect, and may take 3-6 months to reach their maximum effect. These drugs will only have an effect on large prostates, and are effective in about one third of patients. In general, the first choice is an alpha-adrenergic receptor blocker.

Clinical points

- Alpha-adrenergic receptor antagonists are the first choice in the treatment of BPH.
- The drug becomes effective within a few days.
- The alpha-reductases take about 3-6 weeks to have an effect, and may take 3-6 months to reach their maximum effect.

What surgical options are available in the management of BPH?

Presently the main surgical options include transurethral resection of the prostate (TURP) and laser prostatectomy. The main indications for surgery are:

- A poor response to medical therapy.
- Acute retention of urine or a history of retention of urine.
- Bladder calculi secondary to BPH.
- Renal insufficiency secondary to BPH.
- Bothersome lower urinary tract symptoms (LUTS) persisting after medical treatment.
- Patient preference.

Transurethral resection of the prostate still remains the gold standard for treatment of BPH. A specialised telescope, called a resectoscope, is inserted under anaesthesia into the urethra and the overgrown prostate tissue is cut away from inside using an electric current. The urethral lining is removed during this process but it will grow again over several months.

The procedure requires a short hospital stay.

Complications include bleeding, infection, temporary incontinence and dry ejaculations. Late strictures related to scarring may occur.

Minimally invasive approaches with lasers are now being used for benign prostatic hyperplasia.

These include:

- Holmium laser enucleation of the prostate. The holmium laser cuts out the prostate transurethrally which is removed from the bladder using a morcellating tool.
- KTP-YAG laser beam. The laser is absorbed by the haemoglobin pigment in tissue resulting in instant vaporization of prostatic tissue. The bleeding is close to zero despite a generous TURP-like cavity being created instantly. The results of short-term outcome studies are as good as TURP. The advantages claimed by the KTP-YAG laser technique are that there is virtually no bleeding because the laser vaporizes the prostatic tissue and there is no cutting. The patient frequently goes home on the same day, most without a catheter.

Complications are due to damage to the surrounding organs.

Open surgery is still performed for very large prostates (100cm^3).

Progress of the patient

- The patient decides to undergo TURP.
- The postoperative period is complicated by clot retention and a bladder wash is performed. The urine becomes clear on the fifth postoperative day. The catheter is removed and the patient is discharged.

Suggested reading

1. Plante M, Corcos J, Gregoire I, Belanger MF, Brock G, Rossingol M. The International Prostate Symptom Score: physician versus self-administration in the quantification of symptomatology. *Urology* 1996; 47(3): 326-8.
2. Aho TF, Gilling PJ. Laser therapy for benign prostatic hyperplasia: a review of recent developments. *Current Opinion in Urology* 2003; 13(1): 39-44.

Self-assessment

Q1
EMQ

a. Mild elevation of PSA.
b. Increased frequency of micturition.
c. Painless frank haematuria.
d. Nodule on the prostate.
e. Hesitancy.
f. Evaporation of tissue.
g. Tamsulosin.
h. Finasteride.

Select one item from above to match the most appropriate item below.

1. Bladder cancer.
2. A 'storage' symptom.
3. KTP-YAG laser prostatectomy.
4. Cystitis.
5. Alpha-adrenergic receptor blocker.
6. Transrectal prostatic biopsy.
7. Alpha-reductase inhibitor.
8. A voiding symptom.

Q2
SBA

A 70-year-old male presents with difficulty in passing urine, increased frequency, a sense of incomplete evacuation of the bladder and nocturia of 4 months' duration. Abdominal examination reveals no masses. Digital rectal examination reveals a moderately enlarged prostate gland. No nodules are felt.

What is the most appropriate management of this patient?

a. TURP.
b. Laser prostatectomy.
c. Alpha-adrenergic receptor blocker.
d. Alpha-reductase inhibitor.
e. Reduced intake of fluid at night and a period of observation.

Q3
True/False

a. An elevated prostate specific antigen in a patient with symptoms of bladder outflow obstruction is diagnostic of prostate cancer.
b. Nocturia is a storage symptom.
c. Detrusor instability causes voiding symptoms.
d. Holmium laser causes vaporization of prostatic tissue.
e. Retrograde ejaculation (dry orgasm) is a side effect of alpha-adrenergic receptor blockers.

Answers overleaf

Self-assessment answers

Q1 1. (c), 2. (b), 3. (f), 4. (a), 5. (g), 6. (d), 7. (h), 8. (e).

Q2 (c).

Q3 a. (F), b. (T), c. (F), d. (F), e. (T).

Chapter 23

Transient ischaemic attack

Learning objectives

- To learn to evaluate patients with symptomatic and asymptomatic carotid artery bruits.
- To be familiar with the selection of patients with symptomatic and asymptomatic carotid artery stenosis for interventional procedures.
- To understand the principles, advantages, risks and damage limitation strategies of carotid surgery.
- To learn the current status of endovascular treatment for carotid stenosis.

Case scenario

A 74-year-old man experiences a weakness of his right hand while at work and is seen in an urgent assessment clinic. During the episode, he could not write or even hold a pen. The weakness persisted for about an hour and then resolved fully. He has not had any similar experiences in the past. He has a past history of hypertension and ischaemic heart disease. He is a heavy smoker.

He is on nitrates for angina, beta-blockers and aspirin.

On examination, his left carotid pulse is palpable, but a bruit is heard over his left carotid artery. All other peripheral pulses are felt. The rest of the general examination and the cardiovascular and neurological examinations are normal.

The most likely diagnosis: left hemispheric transient ischaemic attack (TIA) due to left carotid artery stenosis.

What is the next step?

- To obtain a duplex ultrasound arterial scan to assess the degree of carotid artery stenosis. The degree of narrowing has a direct implication on the treatment strategy.
- Duplex imaging reveals an 80% stenosis of the left internal carotid artery.

This patient's history is typical of a TIA. However, the diagnosis of TIA can often be difficult because the disability is frequently minor and short-lived and the patient may attribute such symptoms to fatigue. The patient may even fail to bring such symptoms to the notice of a clinician.

The TIA is due to focal embolic ischaemia of the territorial blood supply of the internal carotid artery. This consists of the eye and the anterior two thirds of the brain.

TIAs are characterised by contralateral weakness and/or ipsilateral monocular loss of vision. The latter phenomenon is referred to as amaurosis fugax. By definition TIAs resolve completely within 24 hours.

The typical features of amaurosis fugax are episodes of loss of vision of sudden onset in one eye. The patient describes this event as if a 'curtain has been pulled across his eye'. A part, or the entire vision may be involved. The event is painless and usually lasts for seconds or minutes, but rarely longer than 30 minutes. Amaurosis fugax is believed to be due to temporary embolic occlusion of the ophthalmic artery or its direct branch, the central artery of the retina.

The key issues to be considered to diagnose TIA are:

- Always unilateral (except the speech disturbance).
- Clear presence of a focal neurological event (weakness of the face, arm or leg).
- Complete resolution of symptoms and signs within 24 hours.

Clinical points

- Confusion and dizziness are non-focal symptoms which are almost never due to carotid artery stenosis.
- In TIAs, the loss of vision is ipsilateral (same side as stenosis) and weakness is contralateral (opposite side to stenosis).
- Recovery of clinical symptoms is complete when the emboli disappear by dissolution.
- Carotid artery stenosis, atrial fibrillation and valvular heart disease are possible sources of emboli in patients with TIA.

What is the next step?

- Assess the presence of coronary artery disease, atherosclerotic disease affecting other parts of the vascular system and other comorbid factors before formulating definitive treatment.
- This patient has stable angina. His hypertension is well controlled and he has no diabetes. He is trying to give up smoking.
- The best therapy for this patient is a left carotid endarterectomy.

Why is medical management not considered?

Clinical decision-making in patients with cerebrovascular disease is a question of balancing the risk of intervention (surgery or stenting) with the risk of conservative management (best medical therapy).

What is the risk of stroke?

Randomised trials have shown that the risk of stroke is approximately one in three over 5 years after

TIA in patients with carotid stenosis >70%. However, the risk is mostly in the first few weeks after the TIA so prompt investigation and intervention are vital. The risk of stroke in such patients with stenosis <70% is low, and in these intervention has no advantage over best medical therapy (antiplatelet and statin). Duplex ultrasonography performed by an experienced technologist is a very accurate method of confirming the presence of carotid disease and assessing the degree of stenosis. CT angiography and magnetic resonance angiography (MRA) are the other two non-invasive investigations which can be performed to confirm the severity of carotid stenosis. These two investigations are done when there is a doubt about the results of the duplex scan.

Clinical points

- Surgery is recommended in symptomatic patients when there is 70% or more narrowing of the carotid artery on duplex imaging.

What is carotid endarterectomy?

Carotid endarterectomy is an operation to remove the atherosclerotic plaque which is the usual source of cerebral emboli. Under local or general anaesthesia, the bifurcation of the carotid artery is exposed. A longitudinal incision is made over the common carotid extending to the internal carotid artery to expose the bifurcation. After clamping the carotid artery, the atheromatous plaque is removed and the incision in the artery is closed with a vein or prosthetic patch. This vein can be obtained from the long saphenous vein in the leg and sutured to the edges of the longitudinal incision to make the opening wider. Many surgeons emply a prosthetic patch (Dacron) as an alternative. The main complication of this procedure is a peri-operative stroke.

Several methods are employed to reduce the risk of peri-operative stroke:

- Intraluminal shunting. A plastic tube is placed between the common carotid and internal carotid artery for the duration of clamping for endarterectomy, so that the blood supply to the brain is maintained during surgery.
- Patch angioplasty. As described above, the arteriotomy is repaired with a patch that widens the lumen. In randomised trials this has been shown to reduce the risk of peri-operative stroke when used routinely. It also reduces the rate of restenosis.
- Local anaesthesia. As the patient is conscious during the procedure, the need for a shunt can be assessed accurately by awake testing.

What is carotid angioplasty?

This is an endovascular alternative to carotid endarterectomy. A balloon catheter is placed across the narrowing under radiological guidance and the stricture is dilated. In most cases an uncovered metal stent is then placed across the stenosis to maintain the patency of the lumen. A cerebral protection device is placed in the distal carotid artery during the procedure. This is like an umbrella with a sieve between the struts which prevents any emboli that are dislodged reaching the brain. The device is removed after the stent is in place.

At present, many centres provide comparable results for stenting or open surgery. Stents are expensive. However, there is a subset of patients who are at a higher risk of complications after carotid endarterectomy and they might be considered for carotid stenting.

These include:

- Patients who have undergone neck radiation or extensive neck surgery.
- Patients who have recurrent stenosis after a previous carotid endarterectomy.

A number of randomised trials are under way to determine the exact role of carotid stenting.

What is the role of surgery in the management of patients with asymptomatic carotid artery stenosis?

The benefit of surgery for asymptomatic carotid artery stenosis is much less clear than the symptomatic group. The risks of stroke in these patients are multifactorial. A large randomised trial showed that the risk of stroke after carotid endarterectomy in asymptomatic patients was 6% after 5 years, compared with 12% in the medical therapy group. However, 40 procedures are needed to prevent one stroke. In general the majority of vascular surgeons do not offer surgery or stenting for asymptomatic carotid artery stenosis unless there is a severe stenosis with symptomatic contralateral disease. Some surgeons recommend intervention before major surgery such as coronary bypass.

Progress of the patient

- The left carotid endarterectomy is performed under local anaesthesia. He is discharged home after 2 days.
- At the second clinic visit at 4 months he reports having no further episodes suggestive of TIAs. He has had to quit smoking under pressure from his wife.

Suggested reading

1. Lamont P. Urgent carotid surgery. *Br J Surg* 2007; 94: 921-2.
2. Johnston SC, Rothwell PM, Nguyen-Huyuh MN, Giles MF, Elkins JS, Bernstein AL, Sidney S. Validation and refinement of scores to predict very early stroke risk after transient ischaemic attack. *Lancet* 2007; 369: 283-92.
3. Naylor AR. Time is brain. *Surgeon* 2007; 5: 23-30.

Self-assessment

Q1
EMQ

a. Best medical therapy.
b. Right carotid endarterectomy.
c. Left carotid endarterectomy.
d. Magnetic resonance angiography.
e. Left carotid angioplasy and stenting.

Select the most appropriate next step for the case scenarios described below.

1. A 74-year-old man presents with a history of a classical TIA which lasted for 1 hour, 2 days ago. The duplex scan reveals a 60% stenosis of the left carotid artery.
2. A 70-year-old patient presents with expressive dysphasia which lasted for about 30 minutes. He has had one similar episode 2 weeks ago which lasted for a few minutes. The duplex scan reveals an 85% stenosis of his left internal carotid and a 55% stenosis of his right internal carotid artery.
3. An 80-year-old male is referred with a left carotid bruit by his GP. He is a heavy smoker and has uncontrolled diabetes and chronic obstructive pulmonary disease. A duplex arterial scan reveals a 65% stenosis of his left carotid artery. He is already on aspirin.
4. A 76-year-old male presents with the classic story of a TIA involving his right arm a week ago. He has had a tracheostomy from a previous laryngectomy. A duplex scan identifies a 95% stenosis of his left internal carotid artery.

Q2
SBA

Identify the feature which is unlikely to represent a TIA.

a. Unilateral weakness of the leg.
b. Speech disturbance.
c. Resolution of symptoms and signs within 20 minutes.
d. Confusion.
e. Inability to write.

Q3
True/False

a. Stroke is a complication of conservative management of patients with TIA.
b. Stroke is a complication following surgery for TIA.
c. Stroke is a complication during surgery for TIA.
d. Stroke is a complication during endovascular stenting for TIA.
e. Age, hypertension and diabetes are factors that are predictive of the risk of stroke following TIA.

Answers overleaf

Self-assessment answers

Q1 1. (a), 2. (c), 3. (d), 4. (e).

Explanatory notes

1. The main problem is the risk of stroke. Studies have catagorised patients for stroke prevention based on the degree of stenosis. The cut-off figure is 70%. Therefore, antiplatelet and statin therapy is the best way forward for this patient.

2. His expressive dysphasia is most likely from the stenosed left carotid artery. (Speech is usually controlled through the non-dominant cerebral hemisphere, so in a right-handed man, the embolus is likely to come from the left carotid artery). He has a high risk of developing a stroke because he has an 85% stenosis. He needs a left carotid endarterectomy or stenting.

3. This elderly male is in a high-risk category for complications during and after surgery. Therefore, it is best to re-check the degree of stenosis before any form of interventional therapy. Peri-operative stroke and acute myocardial infarction are two dangerous complications following carotid surgery. This patient is particularly at risk of these two complications because of his reduced oxygen-carrying capacity on account of his COPD and poor peripheral perfusion due to pump insufficiency.

4. This patient who has had a laryngectomy and carotid endarterectomy may pose technical difficulties and is best avoided. He has a high risk of stroke and angioplasty and stenting will be the best option for him.

Q2 (d).

Q3 a. (T), b. (T), c. (T), d. (T), e. (T).

Explanatory notes

A simple risk score, ABCD, has shown to predict 7-day stroke risk after a TIA:

- A - age.
- B - blood pressure.
- C - clinical features (unilateral limb weakness, speech impairment).
- D - diabetes.

The ABCD score is used to predict risk of stroke at 7 days and the California score is used to predict risk of stroke at 90 days.

Many clinicians use the score in clinical practice to triage patients into low (1%-2% risk), moderate (4%), and high-risk (8%) groups.

Patients classified as high risk can be prioritised for immediate assessment and targeted intervention to minimise their risk of future stroke.

The latest addition to the ABCD score is the ABCD2 score which consists of 5 factors:

- AGE 60 or over - 1 point.
- BP >140/90mm Hg - 1 point.
- Unilateral weakness - 2 points.
- Speech impairment without weakness - 1 point.
- Duration:
  - 60 minutes or more - 2;
  - 10-59 minutes - 1.

A total of 6-7 points is possible.

The new ABCD2 can predict the risk of stroke within 2 days after a TIA.

If the ABCD2 score is 6 or more the 2-day risk of stroke is estimated at 8.1%. The risk stratification to mild, moderate or severe may help clinicians to determine whether the patients who have had a TIA should be admitted to the hospital urgently to prevent a stroke.

Chapter 24

Intermittent claudication

Learning objectives

- To learn the initial work-up of a patient with intermittent claudication.
- To be familiar with the investigation of such patients.
- To be able to recognise the indications, benefits and limitations of invasive therapy for limb revascularisation.

Case scenario

A 60-year-old man presents with pain in the right leg of 3 months' duration. He experiences pain in the right thigh and calf after walking for about 100 metres but this resolves after a short rest. He has been smoking 15 cigarettes a day for the last 15 years. He has Type II diabetes and hypertension, but no angina or exertional dyspnoea.

On examination, his pulse rate is 82/minute, the rhythm is regular and BP is 160/90mm Hg. The left femoral pulse is normal to palpation but no distal pulses are palpable below this level. In the right leg, the femoral, popliteal, posterior tibial and dorsalis pedis pulses are not palpable. Doppler examination reveals audible signals in both foot arteries but softer on the right. The ankle/brachial pressure index (ABPI) is 0.6 on the right and 0.8 on the left.

The most likely clinical diagnosis: bilateral occlusive arterial disease.

This patient's symptoms are confined to the right leg, where he has no palpable pulses. The ABPI of 0.6 on the right suggests significant occlusive arterial disease. Because he has no right femoral pulse it is likely that he has a right iliac artery occlusion.

In the left leg, the pulses are absent below the left femoral artery. Although the patient has no symptoms in the left leg, the ABPI of 0.8 suggests the presence of asymptomatic occlusive arterial disease. The absent pulses below the left femoral artery suggest a possible left superficial femoral artery occlusion.

Clinical points

- A history of right leg claudication in a diabetic who is a heavy smoker with absent leg pulses points to peripheral arterial disease.
- A low ABPI confirms arterial disease.
- The ABPI is the most important non-invasive investigation to confirm arterial disease and to assess its severity.

How do arteries become occluded?

The arteries in the body become occluded as a result of narrowings known as atheromatous plaques. The condition is called atherosclerosis. Atherosclerosis is the cause of occlusive arterial disease of the legs, where it usually affects large and medium-sized arteries. The initial event is the deposition of lipids in the intima and media of the arterial wall. The resultant fatty streak is an easily identifiable lesion in early atherosclerosis. Fatty streaks have been detected in children as young as 10. They consist of lipid-laden macrophages overlying the smooth muscle cells of the medial layer. Progression of the fatty streaks leads to the formation of atheromatous plaques.

Healthy normal arteries are lined by smooth vascular endothelium. The development of atheromatous plaques results in roughening of the smooth endothelial lining. This causes turbulence of the blood flow and results in adherence of platelets. Stable atheromatous plaques are well tolerated and may be asymptomatic. For reasons as yet unknown plaques may become unstable. Plaque instability can lead to rupture, with exposure of the lipid core and activation of the coagulation system; platelets adhere to the exposed irregular surface. Plaque rupture can cause occlusion - this is called arterial thrombosis, and is the common mechanism for heart attacks. Platelets that accumulate on a ruptured plaque can detach and embolise and block distal vessels. This is the common mechanism for stroke. Both mechanisms may occur in the legs, where plaque instability can turn a stable stenosis causing claudication into an occlusion leading to limb-threatening ischaemia.

The risk of plaque formation is higher in diabetics because of the associated endothelial and smooth muscle dysfunction seen in this condition.

What is the Ankle Brachial Pressure Index (ABPI)?

Under normal conditions, the systolic blood pressure in the leg is equal to, or slightly greater than the systolic pressure in the arm. When there is an occlusion of an artery, a reduction in pressure occurs beyond it. The Ankle Brachial Pressure Index (ABPI) is the ratio of the systolic blood pressure measured at the ankle to the systolic pressure in the arm. The ABPI is a sensitive marker of arterial insufficiency.

The systolic pressure in the posterior tibial and dorsalis pedis arteries in the feet is estimated by placing a Doppler probe to monitor the signal while a sphygmomanometer (blood pressure cuff) is inflated above the artery. The cuff is deflated and the pressure at which the signal becomes audible is recorded. This is compared with the brachial pressure measured in the normal way. An ABPI greater than 0.9 is considered normal. Values between 0.9 to 0.6 suggest peripheral arterial disease affecting the vessels of the legs. A value less than 0.5 suggests severe, possibly leg-threatening ischaemia.

When the wall of the artery becomes calcified, it becomes relatively incompressible and therefore the measurement of systolic blood pressure in the foot arteries becomes unreliable. This is often seen in diabetic patients with peripheral arterial disease. An ABPI greater than 1.3 is considered abnormal as this suggests calcification of the wall of the artery and a non-compressible vessel.

Clinical points

- An ABPI greater than 0.9 is normal.
- Values between 0.9 to 0.6 suggest occlusive arterial disease.
- A value less than 0.5 suggests severe ischaemia.
- A value greater than 1.3 suggests that the artery is incompressible due to calcification and is considered abnormal.
- The risk of plaque formation is high in diabetics.

What is the clinical presentation of acute limb ischaemia?

Acute ischaemia of the leg or arm is characterised by the six Ps: pain, pallor, pulselessness, paraesthesia, paralysis and perishing with cold. Acute ischaemia is the result of arterial embolism or thrombosis. Paralysis or loss of sensation are worrying signs suggesting tissue necrosis is imminent. Urgent revascularisation within hours is required.

Progress of the patient

- Investigations are performed to:
  - assess the level and severity of the arterial occlusive disease;
  - investigate for concomitant coronary artery and carotid artery disease, as atherosclerosis is a systemic disease;
  - investigate for comorbid conditions such as diabetes, hypertension and dyslipidaemia, which have a bearing on the prognosis both of the patient and their arterial occlusive disease of the leg.

Progress of the patient

- Hb 14g/dL.
- Fasting blood glucose 130mg/dL.
- Lipid profile:
  - S cholesterol 280mg/dL (200-239mg/dL);
  - S triglyceride 240mg/dL (<180mg/dL);
  - HDL 120mg/dL (30-60mg/dL);
  - LDL 220mg/dL (100-190mg/dL).
- ECG - left bundle branch block.
- Chest X-ray - normal.
- The duplex arterial scan dentifies a short stenosis (70% narrowing) in the right common iliac artery and a further short occlusion in the left superficial femoral artery

What is the difference between Doppler testing and duplex ultrasound?

The principle underlying Doppler ultrasound is that the frequency of signals reflected from moving objects such as moving red blood cells shifts in proportion to the velocity of the target (q.v. change in sound of siren as an ambulance goes by). The normal triphasic Doppler velocity waveform is made up of three components which correspond to the different phases of arterial flow: rapid antegrade flow during systole, transient reversal of flow during early diastole and the slow antegrade flow during late diastole. The examination of an artery distal to a narrowing shows characteristic changes in the velocity profile. A monophasic signal is the result of proximal disease, with a delayed rise and decreased amplitude, with non-reversal of flow in early diastole. In severe disease, the Doppler waveform flattens further; in critical limb ischaemia, it is undetectable.

The duplex arterial scan is an excellent first-line non-invasive investigation to assess the structural and functional integrity of an artery. It produces ultrasound images of the arterial tree, but also delineates the changes in blood flow velocity during a single cardiac cycle. Duplex examination of an area of stenosis shows the increase in blood velocity within the artery at that site. The increased velocity is used to determine the degree of stenosis.

Progress of the patient

- This patient has a stenosis in the right common iliac artery affecting the inflow to the leg, causing claudication. He also has an asymptomatic left superficial femoral artery occlusion.
- The patient is referred to a physician. He commences lifestyle therapy.
- He is strongly advised to stop smoking.
- His diabetic control is reviewed and it is decided to continue the same medication.
- His hypertension treatment is reviewed and close monitoring is commenced.
- Statins are commenced to treat hyper-lipidaemia (and to stablise plaque).
- He is advised to exercise within his limitations to improve collateral blood flow.

Why is angioplasty or surgical bypass not considered, to improve the inflow to the right leg?

This patient is not severely disabled with his claudication, although his symptoms are causing significant inconvenience to his lifestyle. Any interventional treatment for occlusive arterial disease can cause complications which can result in the loss of the limb (rare) or even life (very rare). Therefore, the clinician will carefully weigh the risks and benefits with the patient, before considering any interventional procedure. In general, a patient should be severely disabled with the symptoms of claudication, not just be inconvenienced, for an invasive procedure such as angioplasty or bypass to be considered.

On the other hand, as the disease progresses to cause ischaemic pain at rest, digital gangrene, or tissue loss, which are definite limb-threatening situations, urgent revascularisation should be considered for limb salvage.

At present, this patient has no such features.

There is also evidence that lifestyle alterations can result in symptom improvement in a significant proportion of patients.

Clinical points

- Indications to consider definitive limb revascularisation are:
  - disabling claudication;
  - severe lifestyle limitation (e.g. unable to work), if other risks are not unfavourable;
  - ischaemic rest pain;
  - digital gangrene (tissue loss is a limb-threatening presentation).

Progress of the patient

- Six months later, the patient is admitted urgently with discolouration of his right big toe and pain in the right foot which has kept him awake at night for 1 week. He has not stopped smoking.

What is the next step?

- This patient has now developed limb-threatening ischaemia and needs urgent intervention to revascularise his right leg.
- A duplex ultrasound confirms progression of the right iliac artery stenosis which is then treated by iliac angioplasty.

Intra-arterial digital subtraction angiography used to be the standard investigation for peripheral arterial disease. This has now been replaced by colour duplex ultrasound imaging. The main drawback of an angiogram is that it is an invasive investigation with a significant morbidity rate of 1-2%, including distal embolisation, haematoma formation and dissection of the artery. Furthermore, contrast nephropathy is a worry in patients with chronic renal insufficiency.

What is angioplasty?

Angioplasty is a minimally invasive procedure which is done under a local anaesthetic. For iliac disease, the femoral artery of the affected side is punctured, a balloon catheter is positioned across the stenosis under image guidance and it is dilated. A stent may be positioned across the stenosis if necessary. Angioplasty works best for large proximal rather than small distal arteries, and for short stenoses, rather than occlusions.

Why is an open bypass procedure not considered in this patient?

All operations carry risks. Surgical bypass is more invasive than angioplasty. It is usually done under general anaesthesia and therefore carries a higher risk of serious complications such as heart attack, stroke or death.

Progress of the patient

- The patient responds well to iliac angioplasty. His rest pain ceases and he can sleep without narcotic analgesics. He is discharged home after 1 week. He is strongly advised to stop smoking.

Suggested reading

1. Shamoun F, Sural N, Abela G. Peripheral artery disease: therapeutic advances. *Expert Rev Cardiovasc Ther* 2008; 6(4): 539-53.
2. Norgren L, Hiatt WR, Dormandy JA Nehler MR, Harris KA, Fowkes FG; TASC II Working Group. Inter-society consensus for the management of peripheral arterial disease (TASC II). *J Vasc Surg* 2007; 45: S5-67.
3. Scottish Intercollegiate Guidelines Network. Diagnosis and management of peripheral arterial disease. A national clinical guideline. SIGN, 2006: 89.

Self-assessment

Q1
EMQ

a. Lifestyle modification.
b. Angioplasty.
c. Surgical bypass.
d. Aspirin and statins.
e. Amputation.
f. Diabetes control.

Select the most appropriate combination of management for the case scenarios described below.

1. A 60-year-old man presents with intermittent claudication in the right leg for 1 year. He sleeps well. He smokes 15 cigarettes a day, has Type II diabetes, hyperlipidaemia and hypertension. The left femoral pulse is normal but he has no distal pulses. All pulses in the right leg are impalpable.
2. The claudication distance of a 55-year-old postman who is a heavy smoker has now reduced to 50 yards and he is worried that he will soon lose his job. He has hypertension and hyperlipidaemia. He has a non-healing ulcer on his left foot. He is beginning to wake at night due to pain in the foot. His duplex scan shows an occlusion of the entire left external iliac artery and a complete occlusion of the left superficial femoral artery. His left popliteal artery is patent at the level of the knee.
3. A 60-year-old man presents with intermittent claudication in the right leg for 1 year. This has become progressively worse during the last 2 months and now pain in his foot has begun to disturb him at night. He smokes 15 cigarettes a day, has Type II diabetes, hypertension and hyperlipidaemia. All his left leg pulses are absent. He has a non-healing ulcer on the left big toe. All right lower limb pulses are present. The ABPI on the left is 0.4 and on the right is 0.9. An angiogram demonstrates a localised stenosis of the left common iliac artery.

Q2
EMQ

a. Amputation of the limb.
b. Lifestyle modification.
c. Bypass procedure.
d. Common iliac occlusion.
e. Superficial femoral occlusion.

Select one item from above to match the clinical feature given below.

1. Digital gangrene.
2. Rest pain.
3. Simple claudication.
4. ABPI below 0.5.
5. Absent pulses in the lower limb.

Q3
SBA

A 76-year-old male who is on treatment for atrial fibrillation is admitted around 8pm with a history of sudden onset of pain in the right calf since that morning. He complains that his right leg is numb and weak. On examination the right foot feels cold when compared with the left. The right foot is pale with diminished sensation. The left calf is slightly tender and no popliteal and pedal pulses are felt. His right femoral pulse and all pulses in the left lower limb are palpable. He has no chest pain. He is not in atrial fibrillation now.

What is the most appropriate immediate management of this patient?

a. Commence subcutaneous low-molecular-weight heparin and review the response to treatment in the morning.
b. Commence an intravenous heparin infusion and review the response in the morning.

c. Explore the right groin under local anaesthesia and perform an embolectomy and on-table angiogram.
d. Arrange a duplex arterial scan and if an occlusion is found arrange a planned exploration in the morning.
e. Obtain a cardiological assessment to review his treatment of atrial fibrillation.

Q4
True/False

The indications for definitive lower limb revascularisation are:

a. Intermittent claudication.
b. Gangrene of the toes.
c. Ischaemic rest pain.
d. Ankle Brachial Pressure Index (ABPI) of 0.6.
e. Buttock pain.

Answers overleaf

Self-assessment answers

Q1 1. (a, d, f), 2. (a, d, c), 3. (a, b, d, f).

Explanatory notes

1. This patient has simple claudication, and therefore needs no interventional therapy.

2. The rest pain and non-healing ulcer suggest an impending threat to his leg. He has multi-level arterial disease and therefore is not a suitable candidate for angioplasty. The entire length of his left external iliac artery is occluded, as is the left superficial femoral artery. He has good 'run off' with a patent popliteal artery. Angioplasty is unlikely to help him and he needs a surgical bypass.

3. There is a threatened limb loss on account of early rest pain, a non-healing ulcer and an ABPI below 0.5. The localised stenosis is amenable to angioplasty, which is a less invasive procedure than surgery.

Q2 1. (c), 2. (c), 3. (b), 4. (c), 5. (d).

Explanatory notes

1, 2 and 4 are indicative of threatened limb loss and therefore an interventional procedure is justified.

3. No interventional procedure is justified for simple claudication because the procedure in itself is associated with risks. There is evidence that claudicants will achieve symptomatic improvement with lifestyle changes.

5 indicates an occlusion above the femoral artery.

Q3 (c).

Explanatory notes

Acute ischaemia to an extremity is characterised by the presence of pain, pallor, pulselessness, paraesthesia and paresis. The loss of movement and sensation and the presence of local tenderness signify critical ischaemia. These features indicate the need for urgent limb revascularisation, which means an embolectomy to begin with.

Q4 a. (F), b. (T), c. (T), d. (F), e. (F).

Chapter 25

Abdominal aortic aneurysm

Learning objectives

- To understand the pathogenesis of aneurysm formation.
- To be familiar with the risk outcome analysis of surgery for asymptomatic and leaking abdominal aortic aneurysms (AAAs).
- To learn the clinical presentation of a patient with a leaking AAA.
- To learn the management of a leaking AAA.
- To learn the evolving role of endovascular stent grafting in the management of AAAs.

Case scenario

A 72-year-old man is admitted with a 4-hour history of epigastric pain which commenced while he was working in the garden. According to his wife, the pain was so severe that he collapsed while trying to get into the ambulance. He is known to be hypertensive. Eight years ago he had a coronary bypass graft He does not have diabetes, but he was a heavy smoker, having stopped 2 years ago. He takes aspirin and statin therapy.

His first BP recording on presentation to the emergency department is 60/40mm Hg. He looks clammy and pale. He is apyrexial.

The abdomen is difficult to assess because of his obesity. The abdomen is distended and there is some tenderness in the peri-umbilical region. Both femoral pulses are palpable but pedal pulses are not palpable on either side.

The ECG shows no evidence of myocardial ischaemia.

Two 14G peripheral cannulae are placed and 1L of Hartmann's solution started.

During a period of 30 minutes the serial readings of his BP recordings are as follows: 60/40mm Hg, 95/65mm Hg, 100/60mm Hg.

The most likely clinical diagnosis: leaking abdominal aortic aneurysm.

In an elderly man who presents with unexplained hypotension and severe abdominal or back pain, a leaking abdominal aortic aneurysm (AAA) should be entertained as the working diagnosis until proven otherwise.

Inferior myocardial infarction, acute pancreatitis, mesenteric ischaemia, renal calculi and diverticulitis are some of the other conditions which need to be considered. Beware the diagnosis of renal colic in a man over 60!

What is the pathogenesis of an aortic aneurysm?

The strength of the aortic wall relies on layers of smooth muscle, collagen and elastin. The main load-bearing effect is on elastin. Age-related degeneration causes depletion of elastin and collagen, which weakens the aortic wall. The aetiology is related to atherosclerotic vascular disease and the risk factors are the same as for other arterial diseases.

When a segment of the aorta becomes weak, this leads to localised dilation of the segment which is referred to as aneurysm. As the aneurysm enlarges the stress on the wall increases and there is a greater risk of rupture.

Anatomical distortion makes the laminar flow within the AAA turbulent. Most AAA contain a large amount of mural thrombus which may occasionally dislodge and embolise to the distal vasculature.

Most AAA are entirely asymptomatic. Therefore, the clinical presentation is usually related to rupture.

Patients who develop a leaking AAA have a very high mortality. Since many patients die before reaching hospital, the overall mortality is 80%; 50% of those who reach hospital and are fit for emergency surgery survive. Patients with an anterior rupture into the peritoneum seldom reach the hospital. Those with a posterior rupture form a contained retroperitoneal haematoma. The retroperitoneal haematoma produces a tamponade effect which together with hypotension temporarily stops the leak. This is the reason why patients with a suspected leaking AAA in the emergency room should not be resuscitated fully because normalisation of blood pressure may cause rupture of the thrombus.

What is the next step?

- Emergency cross-matching of 10 units of blood is requested.
- An FBC is requested including urea and electrolyte levels.
- A urinary catheter is inserted.
- As soon as the diagnosis is made clinically, a consultant vascular surgeon, consultant anaesthetist, and the operating theatre and ICU are informed.
- If the patient is stable, or the diagnosis is in doubt, an urgent CT scan is arranged on the way to the operating theatre.
- The next of kin is contacted for urgent consultation.
- The CT scan reveals an 8cm abdominal aortic aneurysm with evidence of posterior disruption with a large retroperitoneal haematoma. The neck of the aneurysm is just below the level of the renal arteries. It extends to the aortic bifurcation.

What is the place of CT in the management of a leaking abdominal aortic aneurysm?

An urgent CT is undoubtedly useful to confirm the diagnosis, outline the morphology and identify the relationship to the renal arteries. However, the decision to proceed to a CT depends on the clinical presentation. If the patient is not haemodynamically stable, then a CT scan is avoided in order to proceed directly to surgical intervention.

An urgent abdominal ultrasound scan will identify the presence of the aneurysm but may not always detect a leak. In general, abdominal ultrasound is not favoured by many vascular surgeons as an assessment tool for suspected leaking abdominal aortic aneurysms, since it gives no additional anatomical information.

Aneurysm rupture is an absolute indication for surgery. However, the final decision to proceed with surgery should be arrived at by an experienced surgeon and anaesthetist in consultation with the patient and family.

Many patients with a ruptured AAA are elderly, and pre-existing comorbidities such as advanced cancer, renal disease, and pre-operative cardiac arrest with evidence of cerebral ischaemia make surgery futile.

The next of kin should be involved in the decision-making process about surgery and be assisted to understand the justification for the decision.

Progress of the patient

- In the operating theatre, the patient is prepared and draped before the induction of anaesthesia.
- Rapid sequence induction is performed.
- The surgeon explores the peritoneal cavity via a midline incision.
- The upper extent of the aneurysm is identified and a vascular clamp is applied at this site.
- Distal control of the common iliac arteries is obtained by clamping.
- The aneurysm sac is opened and the haematoma is evacuated. Any back bleeding from the lumbar arteries is controlled by direct suture.
- A tube prosthetic aortic graft is placed, when the iliac arteries are not aneurysmal.
- After the procedure, the legs and colon are inspected for the adequacy of their circulation.
- The patient is extubated before being transported to the ICU.

The purpose of the sequence, preparation and draping before induction, rapid sequence induction and rapid entry into the peritoneal cavity, is to limit the potential effect of general anaesthesia which may cause loss of the tamponade effect by relaxation of the muscles of the anterior abdominal wall.

Progress of the patient

- The patient is managed in the ICU.
- Both feet appear warm and pedal pulses are palpable.
- Good urine output is noted.
- The postoperative period is uneventful.
- He is discharged home after 2 weeks to be followed up in clinic 2 weeks later.

Procedure-specific complications include respiratory failure, myocardial ischaemia, stroke, renal failure, colonic ischaemia and micro-embolism to the legs.

What factors would determine the decision to operate on a patient with an abdominal aortic aneurysm in an elective setting?

The basic principle is to understand the balance between the risk of aneurysm rupture and the morbidity and mortality associated with surgical repair.

The mortality after elective repair of an infrarenal AAA is from 4-8%.

Because of the relationship between the size of the aneurysm and the risk of rupture, the maximum aortic diameter is the main determinant concerning the indication for surgery.

Based on the results of the UK Small Aneurysm Trial, it is known that an aneurysm with a maximum diameter of less than 5.5cm may safely be left and followed up by serial ultrasound to monitor expansion. Most vascular surgeons believe that the risk of rupture escalates in AAA above 5.5cm in diameter, and elective surgery is offered to fit patients.

In patients with significant or irreversible comorbidities, ultrasound surveillance may be continued until the aneurysm reaches a diameter where the risk of rupture outweighs the risk of elective treatment.

Occasionally, AAA may become painful, without evidence of rupture. This is considered a relative indication for elective repair. This is because the pain from an aneurysm is thought to be due to acute expansion, and therefore rupture may be imminent.

Endovascular aneurysm repair (EVAR) is a versatile minimally invasive technique which may become the standard management of abdominal and thoracic aortic aneurysms in the future. Instead of a large abdominal incision, EVAR is done through small groin incisions. A covered stent graft is inserted up the inside of the aorta under radiological control and opened to exclude the aneurysm, thus eliminating the risk of rupture. A significant number of patients who undergo EVAR require secondary procedures to deal with endoleaks or other graft-related problems. The UK EVAR 1 Trial (open vs. endovascular repair) showed significantly lower operative mortality after EVAR than open repair, but after 4 years of follow-up, there was no difference in overall mortality rates between the procedures. EVAR is now recommended by the National Institute for Health and Clinical Excellence (NICE), UK, to be used in selected cases of aneurysm rupture. At present only 50-60% of AAA are suitable for EVAR, but the field is rapidly developing as graft technology advances. The future role of both EVAR and conventional surgery has yet to be defined.

What is the current status with regard to early detection of abdominal aortic aneurysms in the UK?

In January 2008, the Department of Health in the UK announced a national aortic screening programme using ultrasound to cover all men of 65 and above. Men are six times more likely to have an aneurysm than women.

This is the NHS's first men-only screening programme. The national aortic screening programme is implemented using the Gloucestershire aneurysm screening project as a model.

Ultrasound examination screening has been shown to reduce mortality from AAA by 42%.

Clinical points

- Aneurysm rupture is an absolute indication for consideration of surgery.
- Advanced cancer, renal disease, and pre-operative cardiac arrest with evidence of cerebral ischaemia are relative contra-indications for emergency surgery.
- The mortality rate after attempted repair of a leaking AAA is 50%.
- Asymptomatic AAA with a maximum diameter of more than 5.5cm should be considered for elective repair.
- The onset of pain in a previously asymptomatic aneurysm is a manifestation of acute expansion and is an indication for surgery.
- The mortality of elective repair of infrarenal abdominal aortic aneurysms is 4-8%.

Suggested reading

1. http://www.vascularsociety.org.uk/patient/topics.asp.
2. www.nice.org.uk/ip026overview.
3. Powell JT, Greenhalgh RM, Ruckley CV, Fowkes FG. The UK Small Aneurysm Trial. *Ann N Y Acad Sci* 1996; 800: 249-51.
4. Endovascular aneurysm repair versus open repair in patients with abdominal aortic aneurysm (EVAR trial 1): randomised controlled trial. *Lancet* 2005; 365(9478): 2179-86.
5. Earnshaw JJ, Shaw E, Whyman MR, Poskitt KR, Heather BP. Screening for abdominal aortic aneurysms in men. *BMJ* 2004; 328: 1122-4.
6. Cosford PA, Leng GC. Screening for abdominal aortic aneurysm. *Cochrane Database of Systematic Reviews* 2007; 2: CD002945.

Self-assessment

Q1
EMQ

a. Resuscitation, urgent abdominal CT scan and surgery.
b. No surgical intervention, tender loving care.
c. Elective aneurysm repair.
d. Resuscitation in the operating theatre and surgical repair.
e. None of the above.

Select the best practice protocol from above for the case scenarios described below.

1. A 74-year-old male who is known to have a 5cm abdominal aortic aneurysm presents with epigastric pain. His BP is 60/40mm Hg. He looks clammy and pale. The ECG shows no evidence of acute myocardial ischaemia and troponin T is negative.
2. An 82-year-old male, who was brought in with severe epigastric pain and a pulsatile epigastric mass, collapses in the emergency department and has a cardiac arrest. He is resuscitated. He is deeply unconscious and his pupils are non-reactive. His systolic BP is 50mm Hg on inotrope support.
3. A 65-year-old man presents with an asymptomatic infrarenal abdominal aortic aneurysm which has a maximum diameter of 6cm. He is under treatment for hypertension.

Q2
SBA

A 76-year-old male who is known to have a 5cm abdominal aortic aneurysm presents with severe back pain of 1 day's duration. His BP is 170/100mm Hg. The ECG shows no evidence of acute myocardial ischaemia and troponin T is negative. The chest X-ray is normal. A CT scan confirms the presence of a 5.5cm aneurysm without evidence of a leak or any other cause for the pain.

What is the most appropriate next step in the management of this patient?

a. Upper GI endoscopy to exclude a peptic ulcer.
b. Urgent assessment by a vascular surgeon.
c. Management of pain with analgesics and diet.
d. Nil by mouth and a repeat chest X-ray to look for free infradiaphragmatic gas.
e. Discharge the patient on non-steroidal anti-inflammatory drugs and refer to a vascular surgeon.

Q3
True/False

The following statements are true/false with regard to a leaking abdominal aortic aneurysm:

a. It should be considered as the most likely diagnosis in an elderly patient who presents with abdominal pain and fluctuating blood pressure with normal troponin T.
b. The presence of bilateral palpable femoral pulses excludes the diagnosis.
c. Is an absolute indication for consideration of urgent surgery.
d. Mortality following urgent surgery is approximately 50%.
e. The onset of pain in a previously asymptomatic aneurysm is considered to be a possible manifestation of acute expansion of the aneurysm sac.

Q4
True/False

Abdominal aortic aneurysm:

a. Is more often asymptomatic than symptomatic in the population.
b. Is more common in hypertensive patients.
c. May lead to distal embolisation.
d. Of maximum diameter 4.5cm is considered an indication for elective surgery.
e. With a posterior leak is unlikely to reach hospital before death.

Answers overleaf

Self-assessment answers

Q1 1. (d), 2. (b), 3. (c).

Explanatory notes

1. An elderly male has developed a leak in his previously known abdominal aortic aneurysm and is hypotensive. The size of the aneurysm is already known. He needs emergency surgery and resuscitation is best done in the operating theatre.

2. Sudden severe hypotension and cardiac arrest in this 82-year-old man has resulted in cerebral ischaemia which is very likely to be irreversible, as shown by the depth of unconsciousness and non-reacting pupils. The outcome of surgery is very poor. Tender loving care is the best option. The next of kin should be involved in the decision and assisted to understand the justification for the decision against surgery.

3. An aneurysm diameter of more than 5.5cm is an indication for surgery.

Q2 (b).

Explanatory notes

A sudden onset of pain in a patient with an aneurysm indicates possible expansion of the aneurysm. Urgent expert vascular assessment should be requested.

Q3 a. (T), b. (F), c. (F), d. (T), e. (T).

Q4 a. (T), b. (T), c. (T), d. (F), e. (F).

Chapter 26

Thyroid mass

Learning objectives

- To learn the diagnostic pathway of a patient with a thyroid nodule, especially concerning cancer risk.
- To learn the treatment and follow-up of patients with thyroid cancer.

Case scenario

A 76-year-old male presents with a lump in the left side of the neck of 4 months' duration. The patient has recently noticed an increase in the size of the lump. He has no pressure symptoms or symptoms suggestive of thyroid hyperactivity.

His history identifies a previous myocardial infarction in 1995. His recent echocardiogram reveals good left ventricular function. He has no hypertension or diabetes. He is a non-smoker and consumes alcohol in moderation.

On examination he has a visible swelling on the left side of the neck situated in the lower pole of the left lobe of his thyroid gland. No other nodules are felt in the right lobe or in the isthmus. There is no tracheal deviation or cervical lymphadenopathy. Systemic examination is unremarkable.

The most likely clinical diagnosis: solitary left lower polar thyroid mass suspicious of cancer

Thyroid nodules and goitres are not uncommon, the majority of which are benign. The recent increase in size and the age of the patient raises the suspicion of cancer.

The other factors that create a suspicion of cancer are:

- Unexplained hoarseness or voice change.
- Stridor.
- Thyroid nodule in a child or young adult.
- Cervical lymphadenopathy.
- Previous history of neck irradiation.
- Family history of thyroid cancer.

Thyroid nodules, particularly when solitary and clinically obvious, should be investigated, as up to 10% are malignant.

Thyroid cancers are rare in children below 10, but are more common in older children and adolescents. Thyroid nodules are more likely to be malignant in children than in adults.

Differentiated papillary thyroid cancer is the most common type in both children and adults. This has the best prognosis.

Previous head and neck irradiation is a cause of increased risk of thyroid cancer. In fact, nuclear fall-out is a well recognised cause of an increased risk of thyroid malignancy.

A recent change in voice may suggest malignant infiltration of the recurrent laryngeal nerve, whereas it is very rare for a benign thyroid nodule to compress the recurrent laryngeal nerve to cause voice change.

A family history of thyroid cancer is of particular significance in medullary thyroid carcinoma (MTC), which constitutes 5-10% of all thyroid cancers. 25% of medullary thyroid cancers are familial and are inherited in an autosomal dominant manner. MTC can arise as part of multiple endocrine neoplasia (MEN) syndrome.

Clinical points

- High clinical risk group:
  - extremes of age;
  - male gender;
  - history of head and neck irradiation;
  - family history.

In general, papillary thyroid carcinoma has the best prognosis, follicular thyroid carcinoma has a medium prognosis, and anaplastic thyroid cancer has the worst prognosis. Medullary thyroid cancer has a prognosis similar to follicular thyroid carcinoma.

What is the next step?

- Thyroid function tests (T3, T4, and thyroid stimulating hormone (TSH):
  - T3 - normal;
  - T4 - normal;
  - TSH - normal.
- Ultrasound scan. A 2cm x 1.5cm solitary nodule in the lower pole of the left lobe is detected. There are no enlarged lymph nodes.
- The patient undergoes fine needle aspiration cytology (FNAC). This shows a follicular cell neoplasm (T3).

The clinical usefulness of fine needle aspiration cytology (FNAC) depends on obtaining adequate material for diagnosis. FNAC can be carried out without ultrasound guidance when the lesion is easily palpable but FNAC under ultrasound guidance increases confidence that the lesion has been appropriately sampled.

If the lesion is found to be cystic on aspiration, it is important to inform the pathologist whether the lump resolved completely following aspiration. Tumours may present as cysts and any residual mass should be immediately re-aspirated and the specimens identified separately.

FNAC cannot differentiate follicular cell adenoma from a carcinoma because the diagnosis of follicular carcinoma depends on the demonstration of capsular and vascular invasion. Both these features cannot be detected on cytology.

Pathologists usually issue a descriptive report but in many centres numerical coding is added to categorise the diagnosis.

In some cases ancillary techniques such as immuno-cytochemistry may be required.

The diagnostic categories recommended by the British Thyroid Association thyroid cancer guidelines are:

- T (Thy) 1 - non-diagnostic.
- T2 - non-neoplastic.
- T3 - all follicular lesions.
- T4 - suspicious of malignancy.
- T5 - diagnostic of malignancy.

The diagnostic categorisation helps to derive a uniform and comparable plan at the MDT meeting (Table 1).

Progress of the patient

- Results are discussed at the MDT meeting. Although the pathological category is T3, the pathologist raises the possibility of a T4 lesion because of the presence of nuclear atypia and other suspicious cytological features.
- A decision is made to perform a total thyroidectomy and central node dissection.
- A serum thyroglobulin level is obtained.

Why is a CT scan not recommended for this patient?

CT scans are not routinely recommended for diagnostic work-up of all thyroid nodules. They may be useful if the nodule is large or when retrosternal, mediastinal or metastatic spread is suspected.

When a patient has a large nodule with retrosternal extension, CT films are useful to guide the surgeon to plan his operative approach. For example, if the

Table 1. The diagnostic categories recommended by the British Thyroid Association - thyroid cancer guidelines.

Category no	Category type	Plan
Thy 1.	Non-diagnostic.	Repeat FNAC.
Thy 2.	Non-neoplastic.	Two benign results 3-6 months apart is needed for confirmation of benign disease. 'High-risk' patients need a lobectomy.
Thy 3.	All follicular lesions. (30-40%)	Lobectomy. Completion thyroidectomy may be necessary.
Thy 4.	Suspicious of malignancy.	Surgical intervention. Lobectomy/total thyroidectomy decided at MDT meeting. Biopsy for suspected lymphoma.
Thy 5.	Diagnostic of malignancy.	Same as 4.

growth is extending to the anterior mediastinum, a sternal split may be required to gain access. A CT scan also accurately demonstrates tracheal compression and deviation which allows the anaesthetist to plan for a difficult tracheal intubation. A bronchoscope may be needed to guide the endotracheal tube into the deviated trachea.

What is the role of radio-isotope scanning in the management of such nodules? Why is it not performed in this patient?

Technetium or iodine scans are sometimes performed as part of the diagnostic work-up for thyroid nodules as they demonstrate the function of the nodule. However, the initial test recommended for all patients is to establish levels of thyroid stimulating hormone (TSH).

If the level of TSH is subnormal, the patient should have an isotope scan to confirm the presence of hyper-functioning or 'hot' nodules. Hyper-functioning nodules rarely harbour malignancy. According to the American Thyroid Association guidelines, if the hot nodule corresponds to a clinically palpable nodule and if the patient is clinically euthyroid, further evaluation of the nodule with FNAC is not needed.

In general, isotope scans will categorise thyroid nodules into three groups:

- Hyper-functioning nodule (hot nodule). The uptake is more than the surrounding normal thyroid tissue.
- Normal functioning nodule (warm nodule). The uptake is similar to the surrounding thyroid tissue.
- Hypo-functioning nodule (cold nodule). The uptake is below the surrounding thyroid tissue.

This patient's TSH level is normal. Therefore, information gained from an isotope scan will not alter the management.

Clinical points

- The initial test recommended for the diagnostic work-up of a thyroid nodule is to establish the level of TSH.
- All patients with a low TSH level should have an isotope scan.
- Hot nodules need no further cytological assessment if the patient is clinically euthyroid.
- A cold nodule has a higher probability of malignancy.

What is the rationale to perform a total thyroidectomy?

In general, most guidelines on the management of thyroid cancer recommend near total or total thyroidectomy as the treatment for thyroid cancer. The exceptions are the small (<1cm), low risk (well differentiated), intrathyroidal papillary carcinomas.

What is a total thyroidectomy?

The removal of both thyroid lobes, the isthmus and the pyramidal lobe.

What is central node dissection?

Lymph nodes in the neck are mainly classified to central and lateral compartments. The central compartment includes the pre and paratracheal nodes from the hyoid bone superiorly to the level of the sternal notch inferiorly and to the carotid arteries laterally. Most endocrine surgeons include central node dissection as part of a total thyroidectomy. The node dissection increases the risk of postoperative hypoparathyroidism.

What is a near total thyroidectomy?

Removal of all grossly visible thyroid tissue leaving behind the smallest possible amount of thyroid tissue to protect the recurrent laryngeal nerve.

What is a lobectomy?

The complete removal of one thyroid lobe including the isthmus.

Progress of the patient

- Pre-operative preparation of the patient:
  - thyroid function tests are completed;
  - S calcium levels are obtained and used as a baseline for postoperative follow-up;
  - laryngoscopy;
  - the risks associated with total thyroidectomy for cancer, such as hypoparathyroidism and recurrent laryngeal nerve palsy, are discussed with the patient for informed consent.

Many guidelines strongly recommend laryngoscopy prior to thyroid surgery. Pre-operative laryngoscopy must be performed in the presence of voice change and clinically suspected or proven malignant disease prior to surgery. It is also important to have a record of pre-operative status of the vocal cords for medicolegal purposes.

Progress of the patient

- A total thyroidectomy is performed.
- During the postoperative period the calcium level is normal by the second postoperative day.
- Histology reveals an intrathyroidal follicular carcinoma in the left lower pole. The maximum diameter is 2.3cm. Two lymph nodes in the specimen do not show any evidence of tumour. No tumour foci are seen in the rest of the gland.
- TNM classification T2, N0 (refer to Table 2).
- Tri-iodothyronine (T3) 20μg three times a day is commenced as TSH suppression therapy.
- The patient is advised to discontinue T3 therapy 2 weeks prior to the diagnostic pre-ablation scan.

Table 2. TNM classification of thyroid cancer.

- T1: intrathyroidal tumour with <1cm in the greatest dimension.
- T2: intrathyroidal tumour with >1-4cm in the greatest dimension.
- T3: intrathyroidal tumour with >4cm in the greatest dimension.
- T4: tumour of any size extending beyond the capsule.
- N0: no regional lymph nodes.
- N1: lymph nodes present.
- M0: no distant metastases.
- M1: distant metastases present.

Clinical points

- The serum calcium should be checked within the first 24 hours of surgery and subsequently if abnormal.
- A decline of calcium levels during the first 24 hours of surgery is predictive of the need for calcium supplementation.
- Mild asymptomatic hypocalcaemia usually does not need treatment but monitoring is indicated.
- Intravenous calcium is indicated for a calcium level below 1.8mmol/l or if the patient is symptomatic.
- Patients with symptomatic hypocalcaemia must not be discharged without intravenous calcium administration until the calcium level is stable in the preceding 24 hours.

(British Thyroid Association - thyroid cancer guidelines, 2007).

What is TSH suppression therapy?

TSH levels can be reduced by giving supraphysiological doses of thyroxine to patients. Most thyroid cancers have TSH receptors on their cell membrane and respond to TSH stimulation by increasing cell growth. There is evidence that TSH suppression helps to reduce the risk of recurrence.

Clinical points

- The initial dose of T3 is 20μg t.d.s.
- The initial dose of thyroxine is 175-200μg/day.
- The target level of TSH to be achieved is <0.1μg/L.

Most thyroid cancers are TSH-dependent and therefore the suppression of TSH is important. However, this patient will need a pre-ablation scan 8 weeks after total thyroidectomy. The half-life of T3 is shorter than thyroxine (T4), but both will suppress TSH. This is the reason this patient was commenced on T3 instead of T4 after surgery before the pre-ablation scan. Long-term TSH suppression is with T4.

Progress of the patient

- The results are discussed at the MDT meeting.
- The oncologist decides to perform a pre-ablation scan at 8 weeks after thyroidectomy to assess the completeness of the procedure and the need for ^{131}I therapy.
- A small thyroid remnant is demonstrated on the pre-ablation scan.
- The patient is given ^{131}I ablation therapy.

What is a pre-ablation scan?

A pre-ablation scan is an isotope thyroid scan performed after thyroidectomy to assess the completeness of the procedure and the need for ^{131}I therapy. If the scan shows a small thyroid remnant after surgery, the patient is given ablation therapy.

What is ablation therapy?

The goal of this treatment is to destroy any residual thyroid tissue to decrease the risk for recurrent locoregional disease and to facilitate long-term surveillance with whole body iodine scans and serum thyroglobulin estimations.

There is evidence of significant reduction in recurrence rates after ablation therapy.

In general, the majority of patients with a tumour size of more than 1cm in diameter are given ^{131}I ablation therapy.

Clinical points

- A postoperative pre-ablation scan is performed 8 weeks after surgery.
- Thyroid suppression treatment is discontinued 3 weeks prior to the pre-ablation scan and ablation therapy.

Progress of the patient

- The patient is advised to have a diagnostic radioiodine scan (challenge scan) in 6 months and, if negative, 1 year later.
- Serum thyroglobulin estimations should be checked every 6 months.
- If these become positive, a whole body scan and CT/MRI/PET scans are conducted depending on the findings.

What is the role of serum thyroglobulin in the follow-up of thyroid cancer?

Thyroglobulin is secreted by both normal and malignant thyroid tissue. Thyroglobulin levels can be raised in other benign thyroid diseases and therefore it is not useful in the initial diagnosis of thyroid cancer.

Detectable serum thyroglobulin in patients who have been treated with a total thyroidectomy and ^{131}I ablation scan is highly suggestive of residual or recurrent thyroid cancer.

Samples should not be collected for at least 4-6 weeks post-thyroidectomy or ^{131}I ablation therapy.

Serum thyroglobulin is usually checked at 6-monthly intervals following surgery.

Clinical points

- S thyroglobulin is not useful in the initial diagnosis of thyroid cancer but very useful to detect residual or recurrent thyroid cancer after surgery.

Suggested reading

1. www.british-thyroid-association.org.
2. Management guidelines for patients with thyroid nodules and differentiated thyroid cancer. The American Thyroid Association Guidelines Taskforce. *Thyroid* 2006; 16(2): 112-30.
3. Guidelines for the management of thyroid cancer, 2nd edition. British Thyroid Association, Royal College of Physicians, 2007.

Self-assessment

Q1
EMQ

a. Total thyroidectomy and central compartment neck dissection.
b. Thyroid lobectomy.
c. External beam radiotherapy.
d. Radioactive remnant ablation.
e. Radioactive remnant ablation in lieu of completion thyroidectomy.
f. Completion thyroidectomy and central compartment dissection.

Select the most appropriate treatment plan for the case scenarios described below.

1. A 70-year-old male has a solitary 1.5cm nodule in the lower pole of the thyroid gland. FNAC shows an indeterminate cytology and the isotope scan shows a nodule with normal function.
2. A 45-year-old male with a 3cm solitary left lobe thyroid nodule. The isotope scan indicates a cold nodule and FNAC confirms a papillary thyroid carcinoma.
3. A 70-year-old male has undergone a left thyroid lobectomy for a solitary thyroid nodule with an initial indeterminate cytology. Final histology is a papillary thyroid carcinoma with extracapsular extension.
4. A pre-ablation scan performed at 8 weeks after a near total thyroidectomy for follicular thyroid carcinoma shows a small thyroid remnant in a 45-year-old man.

Q2
SBA

Which factor is associated with the highest risk of malignancy in a patient who presents with a solitary thyroid nodule?

a. A past history of neck irradiation in childhood.
b. A hypo-functioning (cold) nodule on the isotope scan.
c. Past history of Graves' disease.
d. The male sex.
e. Past history of subtotal thyroidectomy for a benign multinodular goitre.

Q3
SBA

What is the most appropriate initial investigation that should be performed in a 40-year-old clinically euthyroid female who presents with a solitary left lobe thyroid nodule?

a. CT scan of the neck.
b. Thyroid isotope scan.
c. FNAC and serum TSH levels.
d. S thyroglobulin level.
e. S calcitonin level.

Q4
True/False

a. In the assessment of a thyroid nodule, a thyroid isotope scan is indicated if the TSH level is subnormal.
b. A hot nodule in a clinically euthyroid patient has a low probability of malignancy.
c. Thyroid cysts may manifest as cold nodules in an isotope scan.
d. Cold nodules have a higher probability of cancer.
e. A postoperative pre-ablation isotope scan is recommended at 8 weeks after total thyroidectomy for thyroid cancer.

Q5
True/False

a. A decline of serum calcium levels in the first 24 hours after total thyroidectomy is predictive of the need for calcium supplementation.
b. Mild asymptomatic hypocalcaemia need not be treated with calcium supplementation.
c. Symptomatic hypocalcaemia during the immediate postoperative period is treated with intravenous calcium supplementation.
d. All patients with postoperative hypocalcaemia will need life-long calcium supplement therapy.
e. Symptomatic hypocalcaemia following thyroidectomy is strongly indicative of removal of all 4 parathyroid glands during thyroid surgery.

Q6
True/False

a. Fine needle aspiration cytology provides sufficient information to differentiate follicular adenoma from follicular carcinoma of the thyroid.
b. A Hurthle cell neoplam is recognised with fine needle aspiration cytology.
c. Thyroglobulin is secreted by both normal thyroid tissue and thyroid cancer cells.
d. A raised serum thyroglobulin level is strongly indicative of cancer during a pre-operative work-up of a patient with a thyroid mass.
e. Serum thyroglobulin has a high sensitivity and specificity in the detection of recurrence of thyroid cancer following a total thyroidectomy.

Q7
True/False

Risk factors for thyroid cancer include:

a. Hashimoto's thyroiditis.
b. Familial adenomatous polyposis (FAP).
c. Endemic goitre.
d. Cowden's syndrome.
e. History of neck irradiation in childhood.

Q8
True/False

The features that necessitate an urgent referral of a patient who is found to have a thyroid nodule include:

a. Unexplained hoarseness.
b. Thyroid nodule in a child.
c. Multinodular goitre.
d. Rapidly enlarging painless thyroid nodule.
e. Cervical lymphadenopathy.

Q9
True/False

The following statements are true/false of medullary thyroid carcinoma (MTC).

a. Approximately 25% of medullary thyroid carcinomas are hereditary.
b. Lack of family history does not exclude the heritable disease.
c. High serum calcitonin levels support the diagnosis.
d. The presence of mutation in the RET proto-oncogene implies multiple endocrine neoplasia (MEN) syndrome.
e. Phaeochromocytoma should be excluded in patients who are diagnosed with MTC.

Answers overleaf

Self-assessment answers

Q1 1. (b), 2. (a), 3. (f), 4. (d).

Q2 (a).

Q3 (c).

Q4 a. (T), b. (T), c. (T), d. (T), e. (T).

Q5 a. (T), b. (T), c. (T), d. (F), e. (F).

Q6 a. (F), b. (T), c. (T), d. (F), e. (T).

Explanatory notes

b. A Hurthle cell tumour can be diagnosed by FNAC, but as with follicular neoplasms, FNAC will not differentiate Hurthle cell adenoma from Hurthle cell carcinoma. Hurthle cell neoplasm is a variant of follicular cell neoplasm.

Q7 a. (T), b. (T), c. (F), d. (T), e. (T).

Explanatory notes

d. Cowden's syndrome is an autosomal dominant condition. It causes hamartomatous neoplasms of the skin and mucosa, GI tract, bones, CNS, eyes, and genitourinary tract. Skin is involved in 90-100% of cases, and the thyroid is involved in 66% of cases.

Q8 a. (T), b. (T), c. (F), d. (T), e. (T).

Q9 a. (T), b. (T), c. (T), d. (T), e. (T).

Explanatory notes

MTC accounts for 5-10% of all thyroid cancers. 25% of MTC is familial and constitutes multiple endocrine neoplasia (MEN) 2 syndrome and familial medullary thyroid carcinoma (FMTC). The presence of mutation in the RET proto-oncogene implies MEN2 syndrome.

MEN2 syndrome consists of two types: MEN2A and MEN2B. 2A is associated with phaeochromocytoma and hyperparathyroidism and 2B is associated with characteristic marfanoid facies and mucosal neuromas of the lips, buccal mucosa and bowel.

A comprehensive family history is important. This should include a history of sudden deaths in the family which should arouse the suspicion of occult phaeochromocytoma.

The treatment is a total thyroidectomy. Children with MEN2B should undergo a prophylactic thyroidectomy in the first year of life and children with MEN 2A before the age of 5 years (British guidelines). Life-long follow-up is recommended with serum calcitonin level estimations.

Chapter 27

Hyperthyroidism

Learning objectives

- To learn the clinical presentations and causes of hyperthyroidism.
- To recollect the differences between Graves' disease and toxic nodular goitre.
- To learn the clinical pathway for hyperthyroidism.
- To understand the treatment options and decision making process to arrive at the best option for a given patient.
- To learn the management of hyperthyroidism in pregnancy and those who may conceive during treatment.
- To learn the role of surgery for hyperthyroidism.

Case scenario

A 33-year-old female presents with weight loss despite a good appetite of 3 months' duration. She has become irritable and nervous during this period and is troubled with episodes of palpitations. She is also concerned about excessive sweating which has made her more nervous and depressed. She feels tired towards the end of the day and finds it difficult to carry out fine tasks because of a tremor which she attributes to her nervousness. She has no history of bronchial asthma.

Her primary care physician noticed that she has a small diffuse swelling in the neck and suspects hyperthyroidism might be the cause of her symptoms.

The results of her thyroid function tests show a suppressed thyroid stimulating hormone (TSH) level with a raised free thyroxine (T4) and free tri-iodothyronine (T3) level.

The examination reveals a thin anxious looking female with a mild, diffusely enlarged thyroid gland and slightly prominent eyes. Her pulse rate is 112/minute and regular. She has sweaty moist palms. She has a peripheral tremor.

The most likely clinical diagnosis: Graves' disease.

What is hyperthyroidism?

Hyperthyroidism refers to the hyperactivity of the thyroid gland which produces an excess of thyroid hormones.

The word 'thyrotoxicosis' refers to the clinical manifestations due to an excess of thyroid hormones.

The commonest cause of hyperthyroidism is Graves' disease. Graves' disease is an autoimmune disorder. The condition is characterised by the presence of circulating antibodies (immunoglobulins) to thyroid stimulating hormone receptors. The stimulation of TSH receptors causes hyperactivity of the thyroid gland.

The other common cause of hyperthyroidism is toxic multinodular goitre.

Toxic multinodular goitre is due to hyperactivity of some of the nodules in a longstanding multinodular goitre. For some unknown reason, these nodules have become autonomous and are unresponsive to the TSH feedback mechanism. They function independently and produce excessive amounts of thyroxine and tri-iodothyronine.

Other causes of hyperthyroidism are:

- Toxic adenoma.
- Thyroiditis.
- Drugs (amiodarone).
- Excessive ingestion of thyroxine.

Patients with a toxic multinodular goitre have a nodular goitre which is often large due to its longstanding existence. The surface of the gland is nodular and the enlargement is non-uniform due to varying sizes of the nodules. These patients have developed symptoms of thyroid hyperactivity on pre-existing goitres.

Conversely, neck examination in Graves' disease usually reveals a diffuse, smooth enlargement of the thyroid gland. In general, the size of the goitre seen in Graves' disease is somewhat smaller than in toxic multinodular goitre. Unlike toxic multinodular goitre, the onset of goitre and the symptoms of hyperthyroidism occur simultaneously in Graves' disease.

The striking clinical features make the diagnosis of toxic multinodular goitre and Graves' disease relatively straightforward in the majority of patients with hyperthyroidism. However, diagnostic difficulties may occur in the elderly. The common features of hyperthyroidism in the elderly include anorexia, atrial fibrillation (which is often resistant to digoxin), depression, apathy, heart failure and weight loss.

A suppressed TSH level and a raised free thyroxine (T4) and free tri-iodothyronine (T3) level are typical of hyperthyroidism. But a raised free T3 level can occur with a normal free T4 level, in approximately 1% of patients with hyperthyroidism. This condition is referred to as T3 toxicosis.

A raised free T4 level with a normal or raised TSH level may indicate a TSH-secreting pituitary tumour. This is a rare occurrence.

Clinical points

- Graves' disease:
  - the onset of goitre and clinical features of thyroid hyperactivity occur simultaneously;
  - the goitre is generally uniform in appearance and the surface is smooth.
- Toxic multinodular goitre:
  - hyperthyroidism occurs in a pre-existing goitre;
  - the goitre is non-uniform due to the nodularity.
- Atypical presentations in the elderly may pose diagnostic difficulties.

What is the next step?

- She is started on propranolol 40mg three times a day and carbimazole 30mg daily.
- She is informed that during therapy:
  - her neck swelling may become slightly bigger and her eyes may become more prominent;
  - it will take about 6-8 weeks for her disease to come under control, although she will feel better before this because propranolol will counter the peripheral effects of thyroxine;
  - once the blood tests confirm the euthyroid status, propranolol will be discontinued and the dose of carbimazole will be reduced;
  - a small dose of thyroxine will be added to her therapy at this stage to abort the enlargement of the gland by maintaining the TSH levels within the normal range. The high TSH level is the main stimulus for the gland to increase in size;
  - if she develops a sore throat or any other features of infection she must report to the primary care physician for a blood count and should temporarily discontinue carbimazole.

Beta-blockers are the first choice in the treatment of hyperthyroidism. They are contraindicated in patients with a history of wheezing. This is because beta-blockers block beta-2 receptors of the bronchial smooth muscles and aggravate bronchospasm in asthmatics.

Beta-blockers provide symptomatic relief of anxiety, palpitations, tachycardia and tremor of hyperthyroidism. They also reduce the risk of arrhythmias.

Larger doses of beta-blockers may be required because patients with hyperthyroidism may be relatively resistant to the effects of beta-blockers.

Carbimazole is the most widely used drug of the two anti-thyroid drugs; the other is propyl-thiouracil. The initial dose of carbimazole ranges from 15-40mg a day and the maintenance dose is 5-15mg a day. The drug can be given once daily.

The initial dose of propyl-thiouracil ranges from 200-400mg a day. The maintenance dose is 50-150mg a day. The drug is usually given in four divided doses.

Progress of the patient

- The patient is discussed at the MDT meeting. She has a small goitre and mild to moderate hyperthyroidism.
- Her ophthalmic manifestations are not prominent. Her best option is to have radioactive iodine therapy as the definitive treatment.
- Long-term anti-thyroid medication and surgery should be given as other alternatives.
- At the next clinic visit, the risks and benefits of long-term anti-thyroid therapy, radioactive iodine treatment and the indications for surgery are discussed.
- She is advised to continue the initial dose for 8 weeks until she becomes clinically and biochemically euthyroid.
- She will be able to arrive at the best option for herself after considering all the options for definitive treatment and it will be discussed at her next clinic visit.
- She is advised to report to the clinic in 2 months' time and to make sure her T4 and TSH levels are checked 1 week prior to her clinic visit.

The adverse effects of anti-thyroid medications include rash, fever, arthralgia, headache and gastrointestinal symptoms. If side effects do occur the therapy can be switched from carbimazole to propyl-thiouracil, or vice versa.

Agranulocytosis is rare but if it does occur it usually develops within the first 3 months of treatment. Both drugs, carbimazole and propyl-thiouracil, can cause agranulocytosis.

Patients should be warned to stop the anti-thyroid drugs and seek an urgent blood count if they develop fever, sore throat, mouth ulcers, or other symptoms of infection. Therapy is continued at the initial dose for 4-8 weeks until the patient become clinically and biochemically euthyroid.

Progress of the patient

- During the next clinic visit the patient indicates that she prefers to continue with the carbimazole therapy.
- She is now clinically and biochemically euthyroid.
- She wants to know how long she should continue the treatment.
- She also wants to know the chances of her getting the disease once the medication is discontinued at some stage.
- She is planning to have a baby and is worried about the effects of radioactive iodine if she is to have that option. She is also concerned about the effect of the anti-thyroid medication on foetal development.
- Because she is euthyroid, she is requested to discontinue the propranolol and to reduce the dose of carbimazole to 15mg a day.
- Thyroxine (100μg) is added to her treatment as a 'block-replace' regime.
- She is informed that there is a possibility of relapse after completing the therapy. However, because she has a small goitre and her hyperthyroidism is not severe, she would have a good chance of having a remission after completing the therapy for 12-18 months.
- As for her idea of becoming pregnant, there is no risk to the baby if she conceives 4 months after the completion of the radioactive iodine treatment, if she wishes to take that option.
- She can conceive during medical treatment with carbimazole or propyl-thiouracil. However, the doses of medication must be carefully controlled and kept as low as possible.

What is a block-replace regime?

A small dose of thyroxine is added to the anti-thyroid drug. The purpose of this is to maintain the TSH levels within the normal range. High TSH levels would otherwise increase the size of the thyroid gland.

The optimal duration of treatment is around 12-18 months. However, patients frequently relapse when the treatment is stopped. The patients most likely to achieve remission are those with mild Graves' disease and small goitres. This patient may well achieve a long-term remission. However, anti-thyroid drugs are not very useful to achieve long-term remission in toxic multinodular goitre.

Many endocrinologists use radio-iodine as the first-line therapy (after initial control with anti-thyroid drugs) in the treatment of both Graves' disease and toxic multinodular goitre. It is well tolerated. The only long-term sequel is the risk of radio-iodine-induced hypothyroidism.

The treatment recommended for women who are expecting to conceive during the next 2 years is either radio-iodine therapy or surgery.

What is the place of radioactive iodine for patients wishing to conceive, and during pregnancy and breast feeding?

Radioactive iodine is absolutely contraindicated in pregnancy and for at least 4 months post-partum and during breast feeding. It is vital that patients are fully aware of this and take appropriate contraception to avoid pregnancy.

Radio-iodine can be used in all age groups other than in children.

How does pregnancy affect the assessment and treatment of hyperthyroidism?

In pregnancy, there is an increased requirement for thyroxine. Due to the mild thyrotrophic (TSH-like) effect of human chorionic gonadotrophin (HCG), there may be slightly decreased levels of TSH in the first trimester but it returns to normal during the rest of the pregnancy. Oestrogen increases the thyroid binding proteins in the serum which increase the total thyroid hormone levels in blood, since more than 99% of thyroid hormones are bound to these proteins. However, free T4 which represents the active form usually remains normal.

In the first trimester of pregnancy, normal development of the brain of the foetus is dependent upon maternal thyroid hormones and it is very important that the levels of maternal thyroid hormones are maintained.

How safe are anti-thyroid drugs during pregnancy?

Anti-thyroid drugs cross the placenta. Therefore, constant supervision is essential to keep the patient on the minimum dose required to maintain the patient euthyroid. TSH levels should be monitored every 4-6 weeks and the dose may be further reduced or discontinued 3-4 weeks before delivery to reduce the risks of neonatal complications.

The preferred anti-thyroid drug during pregnancy is propyl-thiouracil because it crosses the placenta less freely than carbimazole. Patients should not be kept hypothyroid during pregnancy but rather in a state of mild hyperthyroidism.

Clinical points

- The duration of anti-thyroid medication is between 12-18 months.
- The majority may relapse at some stage after discontinuing therapy.
- Long-term remissions are mostly seen in patients with Graves' disease who have small goitres with mild to moderate thyrotoxicosis.
- In general, radio-iodine is considered as the first-line therapy in the treatment of both Graves' disease and toxic multinodular goitre.
- Propyl-thiouracil is the preferred drug during pregnancy.

Clinical points

- Radio-iodine is contraindicated during pregnancy and lactation.
- Women can become pregnant 4 months after completing treatment with radio-iodine.
- Men should be careful to avoid fathering for 4 months (life span of a sperm) after completing radio-iodine therapy.

Progress of the patient

- The patient responds to treatment and carbimazole is discontinued after 12 months.
- She is referred back to the clinic after 2 years with a relapse.
- She has not conceived.
- She still will not consider radio-iodine treatment because her next door neighbour's baby has a congenital abnormality. Her neck lump is more visible and this has become a problem for her.
- She now requests surgery.
- She is offered a total thyroidectomy.
- Informed consent is obtained after discussing the benefits of surgery and the risks involved. The risks include early haematoma formation, the possibility of a low calcium level and the need to have calcium supplementation for a variable period of time postoperatively, voice weakness, a very rare risk of recurrent laryngeal nerve damage, postoperative hypothyroidism and the need to have long-term thyroxine.
- She undergoes a total thyroidectomy and has an uneventful postoperative period. She is now on life-long thyroxine treatment.

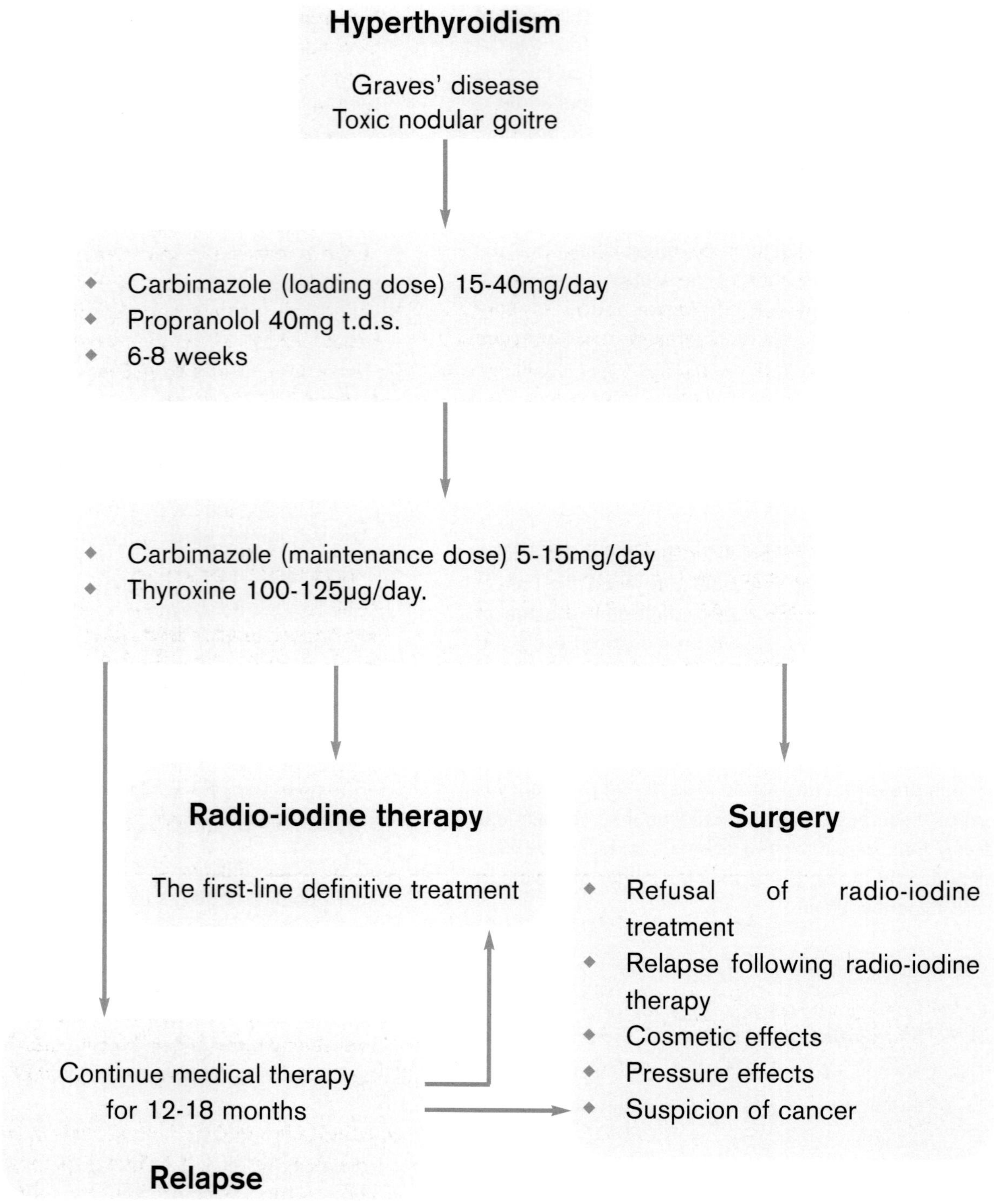

Figure 1. Care pathway for hyperthyroidism.

The two main indications for surgical treatment in this patient are:

- Refusal of radio-iodine by the patient.
- A cosmetically unacceptable goitre.

However, she has no pressure effects and this would be another indication for surgery.

Conventional surgical treatment has previously been a subtotal thyroidectomy with the goal of surgery being to cure the hyperthyroidism while leaving residual thyroid tissue to maintain postoperative euthyroid status. A cuff of thyroid tissue was left behind on either side of the trachea to reduce the occurrence of postoperative hypoparathyroidism. It is also thought to reduce the incidence of postoperative recurrent laryngeal nerve palsy.

However, many endocrine surgeons advocate total or near total thyroidectomy for hyperthyroidism. The reasons for this change of approach are four-fold:

- Firstly, studies have shown that some patients may develop recurrences because the residual thyroid tissue can hyperfunction later. Re-do surgery is associated with a significant risk of recurrent laryngeal nerve palsy.
- Secondly, the potential risk of recurrent laryngeal nerve palsy has changed considerably because of the emergence of the sub-specialty of endocrine surgery with the development of high volume centres.
- Thirdly, the risk of postoperative hypoparathyroidism has reduced due to better surgical expertise and newer techniques of transplantation of parathyroid tissue.
- Fourthly, the development of cancer in the remaining thyroid stump has been recognised on long-term follow-up of patients who have had a subtotal thyroidectomy.

A care pathway for hyperthyroidism is shown in Figure 1.

Suggested reading

1. www.british-thyroid-association.org.
2. Lo CY, Kwok KF, Yuen PW. A prospective evaluation of recurrent laryngeal nerve paralysis during thyroidectomy. *Arch Surg* 2000; 135: 204-7.

Self-assessment

Q1
EMQ

a. Commence propranolol and carbimazole.
b. Offer anti-thyroid medication and reassure that the drugs are very safe during pregnancy.
c. Strongly recommend surgery as the immediate therapy.
d. Offer radioactive iodine treatment and defer pregnancy for 6 months.

Select the best management plan from above for the case scenario described below. Each option can be used once, more than once or not at all.

A young lady accountant presents with weight loss, nervousness, irritability, frequent palpitations and excessive sweating of 2 months' duration. She describes her appetite as excellent. She was planning to come off her oral contraceptive pill to have a baby sometime in the future. On examination she has a mild, diffusely enlarged thyroid gland, pulse rate of 110/minute, sweaty moist palms and a peripheral tremor. Her thyroid function tests show a suppressed TSH level, and a raised free thyroxine (T4) and free tri-iodothyronine (T3) level.

Q2
EMQ

a. Control thyrotoxicosis with anti-thyroid medication and offer total thyroidectomy.
b. Total thyroidectomy.
c. Anti-thyroid medication for 12-18 months.
d. Commence anti-thyroid medication and offer radio-iodine treatment.

Select the options from above that you would recommend for the case scenarios described below. Each option can be used once, more than once or not at all.

1. A 40-year-old female presents with clinical features suggestive of mild thyrotoxicosis of 2 months' duration and a small uniformly enlarged thyroid gland.
2. A 34-year-old male presents with a large toxic nodular goitre with severe thyrotoxicosis. He would like to father a baby.
3. An 80-year-old male who is known to have aortic stenosis, presents with anorexia, weight loss and depression, atrial fibrillation, and moderately high levels of free T3 and T4, and a low TSH level.

Q3
SBA

Which of the following is the first-line treatment for hyperthyroidism in pregnancy?

a. Carbimazole.
b. Total thyroidectomy.
c. Propranolol.
d. Propyl-thiouracil.
e. Radioactive iodine.

Q4
True/False

The following statements are true/false of Graves' disease and pregnancy:

a. Propyl-thiouracil is preferred to carbimazole during pregnancy.
b. Propyl-thiouracil crosses the placenta.
c. The dose of anti-thyroid drug required decreases with the progression of pregnancy.
d. Surgical treatment, if indicated, is best performed during the second trimester.
e. Radioactive iodine treatment is contraindicated during lactation.

Answers overleaf

Self-assessment answers

Q1 (a), (d).

Explanatory notes

Radio-iodine is considered as first-line therapy in the treatment of both Graves' disease and toxic multinodular goitre. According to guidelines pregnancy is considered safe 4-6 months after completing treatment with radio-iodine.

Q2 1. (d), 2. (b), 3. (c, d).

Q3 (d).

Q4 a. (T), b. (T), c. (T), d. (T) e. (T).

Chapter 28

Hyperparathyroidism

Learning objectives

- To learn the clinical presentation of a patient with primary hyperparathyroidism.
- To understand the different types of hyperparathyroidism.
- To learn the diagnostic and therapeutic approach for a patient with suspected hyperparathyroidism.

Case scenario

A 49-year-old male is referred by his primary care physician with fatigue, general malaise and depression of 6 months' duration. His appetite is normal and he has not lost weight. A course of anti-depressants has not helped. He is on antihypertensive medication and his blood pressure is well controlled. On routine screening he is found to have a calcium level of 3.4mmol/L (2.2-2.6mmol/L).

Results of the other investigations are:

- S phosphorus 0.60mmol/L (0.70-1.30mmol/L).
- S chloride 106mmol/L (95-109mmol/L).
- S Na - normal.
- S K - normal.
- Renal profile - normal.
- FBC - normal.
- Urine analysis - normal.
- Chest X-ray - normal.
- ECG - normal except a prolonged QT interval.

The most likely clinical diagnosis: primary hyperparathyroidism.

Hypercalcaemia is the hallmark of primary hyperparathyroidism. Although the differential diagnosis of hypercalcaemia is extensive, primary hyperparathyroidism and malignancies account for 90% of all causes of hypercalcaemia.

This patient has only non-specific symptoms. His renal function is normal. He has hypercalcaemia and hypophosphataemia. This picture is consistent with a diagnosis of primary hyperparathyroidism.

What other leading questions may be useful to support or exclude the differential diagnoses?

- History of peptic ulcer disease?
- History of pancreatitis?
- Bone pain and/or pathological fractures?
- Psychiatric symptoms - depression, psychosis, hallucinations?

These are well described associated conditions with primary hyperparathyroidism. This patient is already under treatment for depression.

- Family history of hypercalcaemia? Familial hypocalciuric hypercalcaemia is a rare condition. These patients have an abnormally high calcium resorption at the renal tubules which is more than 99%. Because it is an autosomal dominant condition, these patients may have a family history.
- History of chronic renal disease? Hypocalcaemia in chronic renal insufficiency will cause hyperfunction of the parathyroid glands and cause secondary hyperparathyroidism.
- History of renal stones? Kidney stones are the most common metabolic complication in primary hyperparathyroidism. This is seen in 15-20% of patients.
- History of malignancies? Hypercalcaemia is the most common life-threatening metabolic disorder associated with cancer. Solid tumours such as lung or breast cancer and multiple myeloma are most frequently associated with hypercalcaemia. The two types of cancer-associated hypercalcaemia are:
  - osteolytic hypercalcaemia which is due to direct bone destruction by a primary or metastatic tumour;
  - humoral hypercalcaemia which is mediated by circulating factors secreted by malignant cells without evidence of bone metastases. One such factor is a parathyroid hormone-like protein known as parathyroid hormone-related protein or peptide (PTHrP). It shares a partial amino acid sequence with normal PTH, binds with the same receptors on skeletal and renal target tissues, and affects calcium and phosphate homeostasis in the same way as PTH.

What is the next step?

- A serum parathyroid hormone (PTH) level is obtained - 400pg/ml (normal 10-65ng/ml);
- An ultrasound scan of the neck is performed. A 2cm well defined nodule in relation to the dorsal aspect of the right lobe of the thyroid gland is noted.

Clinical points

- An elevated PTH in the absence of a familial pattern of hypercalcaemia confirms the diagnosis of primary hyperparathyroidism.
- With the exception of familial hypocalciuric hypercalcaemia which may be associated with a mild increase in serum PTH levels, all other causes of hypercalcaemia are associated with suppressed PTH levels.

A solitary parathyroid adenoma is the cause of primary hyperparathyroidism in 85% of patients with primary hyperparathyroidism. 15% are due to diffuse hyperplasia of the parathyroid glands. The solitary nodule in relation to the right thyroid lobe detected by the ultrasound scan of this patient is very likely to be a solitary parathyroid adenoma. Parathyroid cancers are very rare and constitute less than 1% of all patients with primary hyperparathyroidism.

Clinical points

- Primary hyperparathyroidism:
  - 85% solitary benign adenoma;
  - 15% diffuse hyperplasia or multiple adenomas;
  - <1% parathyroid carcinoma.

Primary hyperparathyroidism is defined as abnormal hypersecretion of parathyroid hormone producing hypercalcaemia and hypophosphataemia.

The increased parathyroid hormone will:

- Increase the renal absorption of calcium and increase the renal excretion of phosphate.
- Promote absorption of calcium from the bone.
- Convert 1:25 hydroxyvitamin D to its active metabolite, 1:25 dihydroxyvitamin D. This will increase the absorption of calcium from the gut by stimulating the formation of calcium-binding protein in the intestinal epithelial cells.

Hypercalcaemia is the hallmark of primary hyperparathyroidism. These patients may have low serum phosphate levels, high serum chloride levels and mild metabolic acidosis. High PTH levels will inhibit the reabsorption of phosphorus and bicarbonate in the renal tubule. Because there is an increased loss of bicarbonate with urine, more chloride is reabsorbed with sodium to maintain the neutrality.

A hypercalcaemic crisis is a rare complication of primary hyperparathyroidism and in advanced metastatic malignancy. The condition is characterised by markedly increased serum calcium levels and an altered level of consciousness or coma.

Progress of the patient

- The patient has a parathyroidectomy.
- Because ultrasound of the neck has detected the adenoma, other tests for pre-operative tumour localisation are not performed.

The characteristic biochemical features of primary hyperthyroidism are shown in Table 1.

Table 1. The characteristic biochemical features of primary hyperparathyroidism.

- Hypercalcaemia.
- Hypophosphataemia.
- Hyperchloraemia.
- Metabolic acidosis.
- High parathyroid hormone level.

The only definitive treatment for primary hyperparathyroidism is parathyroidectomy. In the absence of any major operative risk, all patients with symptomatic and asymptomatic primary hyperparathyroidism are treated with a parathyroidectomy. The rationale for this approach is that the operation relieves the non-specific symptoms and improves survival.

Clinical points

- Parathyroidectomy is indicated for patients with symptomatic and asymptomatic primary hyperparathyroidism.

What are the other methods available for pre-operative localisation of parathyroid tumours?

- MRI may identify the large glands. The sensitivity of MRI is 94% in adenomas and 68% in hyperplasia.
- Selective venous sampling combined with angiography by a skilled radiologist.
- ^{99m}Tc sestamibi scan.

A ^{99m}Tc sestamibi scan is a newer technique in imaging and localization of the parathyroid glands. Sestamibi is a radiopharmaceutical which is bound to the radioactive isotope ^{99m}Tc. This is taken up by both thyroid and parathyroid tissue but sestamibi washes out of the thyroid tissue early after its injection leaving only parathyroid tissue that demonstrates activity at 2-4 hours. ^{99m}Tc-sestamibi is absorbed at a greater rate in a hyperfunctioning parathyroid gland than in a normal parathyroid gland. The test has approximately 90% sensitivity for the detection of solitary parathyroid adenomas.

What is a parathyroidectomy?

In this operation, the surgeon will remove the parathyroid adenoma. He will also obtain a biopsy from the normal glands.

If the findings are of diffuse hyperplasia, some surgeons will remove all four glands leaving half of one gland. Others will remove all four glands and transplant half of one gland to the sternomastoid muscle. Rarely, a cervical thymectomy may have to be performed in case a fifth or ectopic gland is present in the thymus.

Progress of the patient

- During the postoperative period the patient is monitored for calcium and PTH levels for 'hungry bone syndrome'. The postoperative period is uneventful.

What is hungry bone syndrome?

Hungry bone syndrome may follow a parathyroidectomy. The condition is marked by hypophosphataemia and hypocalcaemia that are refractory to calcium and phosphorus supplementation. It is usually seen in patients with longstanding hyperparathyroidism with ostitis fibrosa cystica. The proposed mechanism is a rebound uptake of calcium and phosphorus by bones that have long been starved of these metabolites.

Suggested reading

1. Task Force on Primary Hyperparathyroidism. The American Association of Clinical Endocrinologists and the American Association of Endocrine Surgeons position statement on the diagnosis and management of primary hyperparathyroidism. *Endocrine Practice* 2005; 11: 49-54.
2. Stephen AE, Roth SI, Fardo DW, Finkelstein DM, Randolph GW, Gaz RD, Hodin RA. Predictors of an accurate preoperative sestamibi scan for single-gland parathyroid adenomas. *Arch Surg* 2007; 142(4): 381-6.

Self-assessment

Q1
EMQ

a. Parathyroid carcinoma.
b. Parathyroid adenoma.
c. Chronic renal insufficiency.
d. Sarcoidosis.
e. Metastatic malignancy.

Select the most likely clinical diagnosis from the conditions mentioned above for the case scenarios described below.

1. A 50-year-old male presents with general malaise of 3 months' duration. He has no weight loss or loss of appetite. He is not pale. Abdominal examination is unremarkable. His calcium level is 3.4mmol/L (normal 2.2-2.6mmol/L).
2. A 70-year-old male presents with weight loss, loss of appetite and hypercalcaemia, a low normal parathyroid hormone level and normal renal function.

Q2
SBA

What is the most common metabolic condition associated with primary hyperparathyroidism?

a. Pancreatitis.
b. Osteoporosis.
c. Renal stones.
d. Gout.
e. Nephrocalcinosis.

Q3
True/False

Hypercalcaemia:

a. Is seen in about 10-20% patients with cancer.
b. Is associated with multiple myeloma.
c. Could occur in the absence of bone metastases.
d. Is due to the production of parathyroid hormone by cancer.
e. Intravenous hydration improves symptoms.

Q4
True/False

The following abnormalities are seen in primary hyperparathyroidism:

a. Hypercalcaemia.
b. Hypophosphataemia.
c. Hypochloraemia.
d. Metabolic acidosis.
e. Low parathyroid hormone level.

Answers overleaf

Self-assessment answers

Q1 1. (b), 2. (e).

Explanatory notes

1. Primary hyperparathyroidism and malignancies account for 90% of all causes of hypercalcaemia. In the absence of any features suggestive of metastatic malignancy, a parathyroid adenoma is the most likely clinical diagnosis.

2. This elderly man has clinical features suspicious of malignancy and suppressed PTH levels. With suppressed PTH levels, this patient is unlikely to have a parathyroid pathology. The other common cause of hypercalcaemia is metastatic malignancy and this is the most likely clinical diagnosis.

Q2 (c).

Q3 a. (T), b. (T), c. (T), d. (F), e. (T).

Q4 a. (T), b. (T), c. (F), d. (T), e. (F).

Index